D0122441

AMERICAN HEART ASSOCIATION
FAMILY GUIDE TO STROKE TREATMENT,
RECOVERY, AND PREVENTION

Also by the American Heart Association

American Heart Association
LOW-SALT COOKBOOK

American Heart Association
LOW-FAT, LOW-CHOLESTEROL COOKBOOK

American Heart Association
FAT AND CHOLESTEROL COUNTER

American Heart Association
COOKBOOK, FIFTH EDITION
(also available in an abridged large print edition)

American Heart Association
KIDS' COOKBOOK

AMERICAN HEART ASSOCIATION
FAMILY GUIDE TO STROKE TREATMENT, RECOVERY, AND PREVENTION

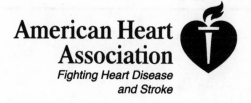

American Heart Association
Fighting Heart Disease and Stroke

LOUIS R. CAPLAN, M.D.,
MARK L. DYKEN, M.D.,
AND
J. DONALD EASTON, M.D.

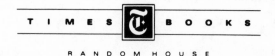

TIMES 𝕿 BOOKS

RANDOM HOUSE

For stroke survivors and their families

Your contribution to the American Heart Association supports research that helps make publications like this possible. For more information, call 1-800-AHA-USA1.

Copyright © 1994 by the American Heart Association

All rights reserved under International and Pan-American Copyright Conventions. Published in the United States by Times Books, a division of Random House, Inc., New York, and simultaneously in Canada by Random House of Canada Limited, Toronto.

Design by Anistatia R. Miller
Illustrations by Hilda R. Muinos

Library of Congress Cataloging-in-Publication Data

Caplan, Louis R.
   American Heart Association family guide to stroke treatment,
recovery, and prevention / Louis R. Caplan, Mark L. Dyken, J. Donald
Easton.—1st ed.
          p.   cm.
   Includes index.
   ISBN 0-8129-2011-2
   1. Cerebrovascular disease—Popular works.   I. Dyken, Mark L.
II. Easton, J. Donald.   III. American Heart Association.   IV. Title.
RC388.5.C329   1993
616.8′1—dc20   92-50500

Manufactured in the United States of America

9   8   7   6   5   4   3   2

First Edition

Acknowledgments

The mission of the American Heart Association is to reduce death and disability from cardiovascular diseases and stroke. To help accomplish this we decided to produce this *Family Guide to Stroke*. Many American Heart Association volunteers and staff were involved in this effort. This book exists today because of their dedication to our mission and to this project.

One of the key people involved in this project was William H. Thies, Ph.D., AHA Science Consultant. He spearheaded the team and paid keen attention to the scientific details of the book.

Three AHA volunteers provided the expertise that was the basis for the text and illustrations. Louis R. Caplan, M.D., Mark L. Dyken, M.D., and J. Donald Easton, M.D., devoted countless hours and careful attention to this project.

Our managing editor, Jane Ruehl, orchestrated the writing, editing, and production of the book. Cheryl Bates, Consumer Publications Consultant, managed the project and kept the numerous lines of communication open. Sarah Trotta was the writer who actually transformed the words of the experts into eminently readable text. Special thanks go to Pat Kasell for insightful manuscript review and to Gerre Gilford and Debra Bond for skillful word processing.

The talents of all these people came together to create the book you see before you. We are grateful for their efforts and proud of the book we offer as practical help to all of you whose lives have been touched by stroke.

Rodman Starke, M.D.
Senior Vice President
Office of Scientific Affairs
American Heart Association,
National Center

Contents

Introduction

I f you are reading this book, chances are you or a loved one has had a stroke or the warning signs of one. Stroke is a frightening event—for those experiencing it and for their families. You want to know more about what has happened, what to expect, and how to cope. It's likely that you never heard or thought too much about stroke before. Yet stroke is the number-one cause of serious disability in the United States. It is the third most common cause of death, behind only heart disease and cancer. More than one-fourth of all strokes happen to people below age sixty-five. Strokes are obviously extremely serious illnesses, real medical emergencies. Whether you or a loved one has had a stroke, you want to know what is in store. That's where this book comes in. It's written for stroke survivors, families whose lives have been touched by stroke, and those who are at risk for stroke.

The statistics show us that stroke is far too common in our society. But there is more to the story. Much is being done to reduce stroke's often disastrous effects. More people than ever before survive stroke each year. In fact, stroke deaths have fallen to half of what they were as recently as 1972. Doctors today know much more about the mechanics of stroke. Better treatment strategies and rehabilitation and recovery therapies have been developed over the past generation. All these things put together are believed to account for some of the incredible improvement in stroke survival—but not all of it. Doctors are convinced that "preventive medicine" has been the most effective means of reducing the likelihood of stroke. That's terrific news, because it confirms the notion that each of us has a great deal of control over our own health—much more than we used to assume.

The Importance of Preventive Medicine

What is "preventive medicine" for stroke? Basically, it begins with identifying the risk factors in our personal health profile that may predispose us to stroke or other associated disease. Then we must change our lifestyles to reduce or eliminate those factors. This idea has caught on very successfully where heart disease is concerned. Today most people know that they can help their hearts and live longer by getting regular exercise, eating right, seeing a doctor regularly, and not smoking. They can identify the warning signs of a heart attack and are aware that they should go to the hospital as soon as those signs appear. This knowledge has helped reduce death from cardiovascular disease by almost a third in the decade between 1980 and 1990.

Well, today doctors have identified similar risk factors and warning signs for stroke—and they are just as important to your health. But many people don't yet know what those risk factors and warning signs are, or what to do about them. Part of the mission of this book is to help you identify those factors that put you at personal risk of stroke. You can then work with your doctor to eliminate them from your own health profile, or at least reduce their effect.

Take high blood pressure, or hypertension, for example. High blood pressure is the single most important risk factor for stroke over which an individual has some control. Over time, high blood pressure injures blood vessels and vital organs in the body. When high blood pressure coexists with other undesirable conditions, such as heart disease, diabetes, or obesity, it becomes even more dangerous. High blood pressure is easy to detect in a simple test at a doctor's office, and it's relatively easy to control. Yet more than 63 million Americans suffer from the condition—and almost half of them don't even realize it. Four out of ten Americans who are aware of their hypertension don't take adequate care to bring it under control.

Cigarette smoking is another dire but completely preventable risk factor for stroke (as well as other disease). Fortunately, fewer and fewer people in this country smoke. It is believed that this fact has contributed greatly to the recent overall drop in heart disease and stroke deaths. Yet about 46 million people still do smoke—and that's 46 million who are at a needlessly greater risk of stroke, heart disease, and cancer. If you smoke, stop! In only a year, your risk of stroke begins to drop. Within ten years, your risk is virtually what it would have been if you had never smoked. It's that simple.

Other stroke risk factors, such as your age, can't always be modi- fied or eliminated. With your doctor, consider your own risk factors carefully. See which of them you might eliminate or reduce. And then do so. If you have already had a stroke, you *can* help reduce the likelihood of having a second stroke. Identify those habits you can change or health concerns you can remedy that will help you reduce your risk. Don't think that you are ever "too old" to benefit from making this important effort. Even if you are a lifelong smoker or haven't exercised since you were in high school, don't despair. Your health will improve if, for example, you stop smoking now or take up some appropriate form of regular exercise (under a doctor's supervision). It is never too late to improve your health.

Your mother probably told you that "an ounce of prevention is worth a pound of cure." That maxim could have been coined by health care professionals. They would be the first to tell you that no doctor's remedy after the fact will ever be as beneficial as following practices that can prevent a stroke from happening in the first place. But it's really up to you. Resolve to do whatever it takes. Learn everything about your condition that you can. Your doctor will help. So can this book. If you've had a transient ischemic attack or other warning sign, you can take steps that will reduce your risk of suffering a full-blown stroke. And if you've already had a stroke, you can improve your odds of not having another. At the very least, taking care of your risk factors has been shown to change the type of stroke you may have. People who manage and modify their risk factors tend to have milder strokes. They also tend to suffer fewer of the more damaging hemorrhagic strokes than others.

Involve your family. Often family members share the same habits and can benefit from making the lifestyle changes you are making. And you can support each other at the same time.

Improvements in Stroke Treatment and Recovery

By zeroing in on the risk factors for stroke, researchers have contributed greatly to our ability to prevent stroke. This has helped make possible the general downward slide in overall stroke incidence in this country. Major medical and diagnostic break-throughs have been made recently, and developments can be expected to continue. Elsewhere, noninvasive tests are giving doctors increasingly clearer pictures of the brain and its blood vessels without resorting to surgery. These developments and others are making stroke treatment ever more effective.

Most people who have had a stroke are worried about what kind of recovery to expect. Be assured that modern stroke care is very much involved with preserving as much function as possible, as soon as possible. More than three million living Americans have had a stroke. Many of them have been rehabilitated successfully. Some people have even gone on to do some of their best work after a stroke. Famous examples of this include the actress Patricia Neal and President Dwight D. Eisenhower. Today we know that the sooner rehabilitation begins, the better. In fact, this activity starts right at the patient's bedside.

Not all people who have had strokes need such rehabilitation, however. Despite a reputation for it, most strokes are not completely incapacitating. Some people recover completely, while others are left with only mild deficits. Even those who have been severely handicapped by their strokes can often be taught to walk and care for themselves again and to remain independent.

Timing Is Everything

Traditionally, stroke has resisted a "cure." Until recently, doctors didn't have access to the kinds of diagnostic tools that could tell them precisely what was wrong, or where. Drugs didn't exist that could prevent or interrupt a stroke. Because of all this, stroke was very much a "watch and wait" illness.

But that was then. Today researchers are closer than ever to releasing new clinical therapies that will allow doctors to intervene during a stroke and interrupt brain tissue destruction. Even current treatments can help prevent some loss of brain tissue and improve the odds of survival itself. But they must be administered shortly after a stroke begins. **For a person who is having a stroke, the key to benefiting from these developments is to get to a hospital as soon as possible!**

Today doctors can take a number of steps to help prevent a

full-blown stroke from occurring—provided they are given enough advance warning. Fortunately, many strokes give small warnings before they start in earnest. Those warning symptoms are listed on page 37. You and your loved ones should learn these warning signs by heart.

Reason for Hope

Having a stroke is a traumatic experience, and coping with it is hard. But these days there are many reasons to feel hopeful about stroke care and prevention. We know more than ever before about how to reduce the risk of suffering a first or second stroke. And we know the warning signs of impending stroke. These signs can mean the difference between a mild stroke or a severe one, or even between a stroke or no stroke at all. Stroke diagnosis and treatment are more advanced today than ever before. Experimental therapies show promise for minimizing brain damage from some strokes—if started early enough.

You've had a stroke, or the warning signs of one, but that isn't the end of the story. You have a lot to do now—work with your doctor to help speed your recovery and learn about your condition. Work with therapists to learn new skills, and work to modify or eliminate your risk factors for stroke. Not all of it will be easy or fun. But your willpower and your determination will help you. And so will learning more about stroke. Equally important is the support of caring friends and family. All these things together will help put you back in control of your life, and that *does* feel good.

Dealing with the aftermath of strokes is what the American Heart Association's Stroke Connection is all about.

The Stroke Connection, formerly known as the Courage Stroke Network, was started in 1979 by a group of stroke survivors and caregivers. Its mission: To provide a forum for stroke survivors, their family members, and the professionals who serve them, to share information and experiences related to living with stroke.

In August 1993, to further expand on the American Heart Association's mission to reduce disability and death from cardiovascular diseases and stroke, the AHA assumed the responsibility for the activities previously conducted by the Courage Stroke Network.

Currently, there are over 850 stroke groups nationwide that

serve more than 45,000 stroke survivors, caregivers, and professionals. There are also groups and connections in several foreign countries.

For questions about this valuable service to stroke survivors, caregivers, and the health professionals who serve them, contact the AHA Stroke Connection at 1-800-553-6321.

Most of this book is written directly to the stroke survivor. Usually, the "you" in the text is the person who has survived a stroke. There are a few exceptions to this. For instance, in Chapter Six we discuss adapting the home for those with disabilities. The "you" in that case is the person making the necessary changes. In the text, we often use examples of unidentified stroke patients and the professionals who treat them. To make the book easier to read, we tried to avoid the cumbersome "he or she" and "him or her." Instead we sometimes use the masculine form and sometimes the feminine form.

We have also included fictionalized stories of people coping with stroke. These accounts, based on doctors' encounters with stroke survivors, offer a glimpse of the human side of the stroke experience. They illustrate how others who have had strokes have met the challenge. Reading them may inspire you to cope as well.

The information in this book is intended to help you understand stroke. Please do not use it to try to diagnose or plan treatment for individuals. Only a doctor can diagnose and prescribe treatment. We hope this book will help you form a more effective partnership with your doctor as you plan together for a healthier future.

AMERICAN HEART ASSOCIATION
FAMILY GUIDE TO STROKE TREATMENT, RECOVERY, AND PREVENTION

1
The Warning Signs of Stroke

A s the name implies, stroke seems to be a force of nature that hits without warning—a real bolt from the blue. But it isn't, really. In most cases, stroke results from the accumulation of a lifetime's worth of daily habits, a collection of small insults that have finally added up to a major event. For a smaller number of people, stroke results from years of wear and tear on a blood vessel with a weak spot.

No matter the cause, stroke is always a traumatic event for the people it affects—and about 500,000 Americans alone experience a stroke each year. Many are surprised to learn that of this number, over 145,000 people die. That makes stroke this country's third-highest killer, behind only heart disease and cancer.

But these numbers tell just part of the story. About 69 million Americans have one or more forms of heart and blood vessel disease.

Stroke is clearly a very serious subject. It's a medical emergency, a life-threatening, frightening development we'd all choose to do without. Yet any of the warning signs for stroke can serve to snap us to attention. They can help motivate us to change some of those habits we've always meant to improve or get rid of. We may also

1

change some habits that we didn't know were detrimental to our health. We do each have some control over whether we have a first stroke or are likely to have a second one.

Harry had just left the dinner table to watch the early evening news with his wife when a strange thing happened. No sooner had he picked up the television remote control to change channels than it tumbled out of his right hand. At the same time, his right leg became weak under his weight, and he found he had to sit down.

Harry was alarmed. For a minute he thought he was having a heart attack, because he did have a heart condition. But he felt no pain. He wondered why his hand suddenly seemed to have a mind of its own.

When Janet saw her husband drop the remote control and start to lose his balance, she quickly asked him what was wrong. Harry's speech was slurred and he had difficulty answering. Janet knew her husband was showing some of the classic signs of stroke. She also knew she couldn't waste a moment. She went straight to the phone and called for an ambulance to take her husband to the hospital.

At the emergency room, the admitting staff was waiting for Harry. They administered several tests right away. Those tests and the doctor's exam proved that Harry had had an occlusive stroke, the result of a blocked vessel.

Thanks to Janet's decisive action, the medical staff at the hospital began Harry's treatment very soon after the onset of his stroke. Their immediate attention contributed to his positive recovery outlook.

Fortunately, Harry's stroke left him with only limited physical impairments. By the time he left the hospital, he was already in physical therapy, and he continued to improve. Harry and Janet joined a stroke club where they met weekly to talk with other stroke survivors about their experiences. At the same time, Harry's doctor was actively treating his heart condition to help prevent future stroke.

People who have had a stroke can begin to establish better, more healthful habits immediately—and to feel the benefits almost as quickly. And the benefits are real whether you have already had a stroke or you've noticed some of the warning signs of one. You can significantly reduce your risk of a second or initial stroke by adopting a more healthful lifestyle now. This is true no matter what your previous habits were or how long you maintained them. You can greatly reduce your future risk of stroke by controlling related medical problems, such as high blood pressure and heart disease, and stopping smoking. It is also quite possible that a leaner diet and more exercise could have a favorable effect. We'll discuss these important goals later in this book.

Let's begin by taking a closer look at what happened to cause a stroke in the first place.

What Is a Stroke?

A general discussion of stroke really begins with a look at the brain, the stage upon which everything takes place.

The brain is the most complex organ of the human body and one in which different areas carry out specialized functions. The average brain weighs just under three pounds. An amazing collection of nerve cells, or neurons, it is responsible for all the signals and sensations that allow us to think, move, and react. This vast network of nerve cells communicates with itself as well as with the rest of the body in order to do its complicated, delicate job.

Not surprisingly, the brain requires a lot of energy to keep it running. Yet despite this tremendous requirement, the brain is the only organ in the body that can't store energy for consumption later. It requires a constant supply of oxygen and nutrients. It gets these from blood, circulated twenty-four hours a day from the heart through the arteries to the brain and other areas of the body. Despite its relatively small size, fully one-fourth of all the blood pumped by the heart finds its way into the brain. When that blood supply falters, a stroke occurs in the affected part of the brain. Where the stroke occurs and how large it is determines the extent and type of brain damage that results. Some people who have a stroke are diagnosed and treated by their regular doctors, others are treated by stroke experts. Often, such experts are neurologists, doctors who are trained to treat problems of the brain. The symptoms of stroke may appear anywhere in the body—a weak or paralyzed leg or an inability to speak, for instance. But these symptoms really indicate neurologic damage to the part of the brain that controls those movements and activities. For a clear idea of how the brain works, let's get better acquainted with the brain and what it does.

The Brain: Where Strokes Happen

A stroke occurs when one of the arteries carrying nutrients and oxygen to the brain either becomes clogged or ruptures. Stroke can be a particularly confusing event to understand because the symptoms of stroke are easily mistaken for the problems themselves. For example, with stroke, a paralyzed arm or the inability to see to one side is not what it may appear to be. These symptoms do not indicate a problem in the muscles or bones of the arm—the arm itself is fine. They do not suggest a vision problem in the eyeball—the eyeball upon examination looks normal. In both of these stroke cases, and others, the problem lies in the brain itself. Because of damage to the brain tissue, the brain simply is unable to give directions to the arm in the first case or to interpret the signals being sent from the eyeball in the second.

Physicians carefully evaluate a patient's symptoms and run tests so they can accurately determine which part of the brain was affected by the stroke. This is possible because, as we'll see, the brain is a highly specialized organ, with different areas largely responsible for different jobs. After all, the brain has an awful lot to do! It controls everything that happens in the body. The way we move, feel, perceive, behave, and think is the result of decisions made in the brain. Even our emotions are directed from the brain. Some of these behaviors are voluntary. For example, we think before we speak (usually). Some actions are involuntary—done without thinking first. We pull our hand quickly away from a flame or get goose pimples if we aren't dressed warmly enough on a cool spring day. By separating these diverse responsibilities into different areas, the brain is able to achieve a degree of complexity in its operation that is truly breathtaking. But this complexity, along with the fact that when brain cells die, they are never replaced, can also make the brain extremely sensitive to the smallest injuries.

Understanding something of the way in which the brain is organized is important to understanding why strokes have the effects they do. It's time for a brief tour.

A Map of the Brain

About the size and shape of your two fists pressed together at the palms, the brain looks something like a soft, wrinkled walnut that sits in the skull at the top of the spinal cord. With the spinal cord, the brain makes up the body's **central nervous system, or CNS.** The central nervous system collects incoming signals, sorts them, and then sends them along to the brain for "processing." Reporting to the CNS is the **peripheral nervous system.** This collection of nerves, rather like a freeway system, fans outward from the spinal column to reach everything from the fingertips to the heart to the muscles of the calves. Together these systems carry a tremendous amount of information back and forth between the brain and the rest of the body.

Each nerve is made up of bundles of nerve fibers. Nerve cells, called **neurons,** communicate with each other, sending and receiving messages in a kind of electrical relay between the brain and chosen end points in the body. **Sensory nerve fibers** send information to the brain. **Motor nerve fibers** carry instructions from the central nervous system to the muscles. The brain can also affect activities in the body chemically, by triggering a release of **hormones** into the bloodstream. Hormones are produced in the **endocrine glands** and are controlled by the brain.

Writers Robert Ornstein and Richard F. Thompson have compared the structure of the brain to a ramshackle old house that is periodically added on to without destroying any of the original structure. If we add on a more modern family room, for example, we tend to use the old one less, although it is still good for some jobs. So it is with the brain. As it has evolved over thousands and thousands of years, some of the jobs originally done by the oldest parts of the brain have been taken over and improved upon by the newer areas. We still use the old parts for some things, but we have also developed new needs that the newer part of the brain is better adapted to satisfy. This partially explains why a stroke involving one area of the brain can have such a different effect on a person than a similar-size stroke involving another area. Let's look at each area separately, starting with the original part of the brain.

The Brain Stem

Not surprisingly, the oldest part of the brain lies at the top of the spinal cord. Sometimes called the "reptilian brain" because it is so primitive, the **brain stem** is really an extension of the spinal cord. The brain stem includes the **medulla,** the **pons,** and the **midbrain.** The medulla is responsible for regulating those involuntary processes of the body that keep us going. Breathing, swallowing, blood pressure, and heart rate are all monitored from here. The medulla is also the place through which all the nerve fibers going from the cerebral cortex to the spinal cord must pass. The pons, which means "bridge," links the back of the brain to the upper portions, allowing them to communicate with each other. Strokes in the brain stem are often fatal. When they aren't, they often interfere with functions we think of as being automatic, such as swallowing.

Thalamus, Hypothalamus, and Pituitary Gland

At the top of the brain stem and underneath the limbic system are the thalamus, hypothalamus, and pituitary gland. The **thalamus** is the staging area for all information headed to the cerebral hemispheres. It presorts a lot of the information and directs it to the proper portion of the cerebral hemispheres—in much the same way that a good secretary will troubleshoot for the boss. A stroke in this area can result in profound sensory loss and sometimes unusual pain syndromes. The **pituitary gland** regulates the body through chemical reactions (rather than electrical ones) by monitoring the release of certain hormones into the bloodstream. The **hypothalamus,** a very tiny part of the brain, controls some of its most important functions. Whether we sleep, eat, make love, maintain a steady body temperature—or a number of other basic survival functions—depends on the say-so of this little part of the brain. Strokes do sometimes occur in these areas.

The Cerebellum

Located at the back of the brain and looking a bit like a pillow for the back of the cerebrum lies the **cerebellum,** or "little brain." It is also responsible for a number of our automatic responses and behaviors. With the **basal ganglia,** which it is near, the cerebellum helps modulate body movements. It helps monitor and maintain a sense of balance and coordination, and it stores the memory of muscle movements that have become habit. A stroke involving this area could result in a lack of coordination, clumsiness, shaking, or other muscular difficulties.

The Limbic System

Tucked beneath the overarching cerebrum and above the midbrain lies the area known as the **limbic system.** Like the brain stem below it, the limbic system maintains some of our basic bodily functions automatically. But it also is involved with those kinds of responses that have to do with survival. Sexual drive, the "fight or flight" response to threatening situations, and hunger all find root in the limbic system deep within the brain. Strokes are unusual here, but when they occur they can either inhibit these drives or cause a person to lose all natural inhibitions.

The Cerebrum

Our tour has led us gradually upward from the brain stem, culminating with literally the crowning glory of the brain—the **cerebrum.** Here is the part of the brain we think of as most distinctly human. And we should: The cerebrum is much more highly developed in man than in any other animals. The cerebrum receives incoming information, analyzes it, compares it with other information it has stored in the past, and decides what to do next. If action is required, it sends instructions to the appropriate muscles. The cerebrum is where we decide to reach out and hug a friend, to think about art or mathematics, store memories—all sorts of perfectly average and yet extraordinary things. Because the cerebrum is so complex, it deserves an expanded explanation. Unfortunately, it is a common site for stroke damage of one kind or another, and that also makes it worth looking at carefully here.

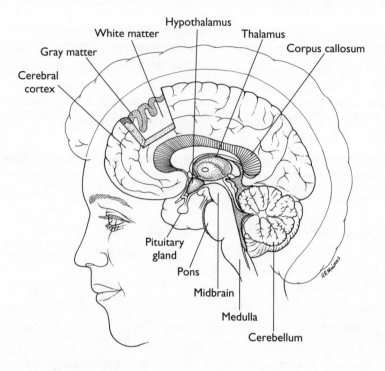

This cross-sectional view of the brain identifies many of its most important parts.

Two Hemispheres

The cerebrum is divided into two similar halves, like many parts in our bodies. These halves, called the **cerebral hemispheres,** govern the opposite sides of the body. The left hemisphere, for example, sends messages to and receives messages from the right side of the body. The right hemisphere does the same thing for the left side of the body. The two halves of the cerebrum communicate with each other across a dense network of nerve fibers that connect them deep inside the brain. This network is called the **corpus callosum.**

Why have two hemispheres that direct the activities of the opposite sides of the body? As it happens, this is a good survival technique. While each hemisphere specializes to some extent in the tasks it does, it can also compensate for the other hemisphere if necessary, most easily in the childhood years. (The theory is that this protects the mental development of children who may suffer head trauma during birth.) The point is, the differences between

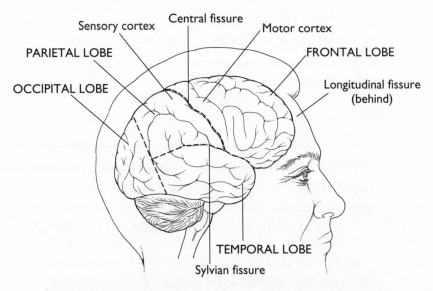

Sensory cortex · Central fissure · Motor cortex · PARIETAL LOBE · FRONTAL LOBE · OCCIPITAL LOBE · Longitudinal fissure (behind) · TEMPORAL LOBE · Sylvian fissure

The cerebrum is the seat of voluntary movement, rational thought, and emotions. It is divided into roughly equal halves. Because it is so big and does so many different jobs, the cerebrum is commonly discussed in terms of four separate areas, or lobes. Three particularly deep wrinkles in the brain's cerebral cortex form the artificial boundaries for these areas and help identify them for doctors. They are the longitudinal fissure, the central fissure, and the Sylvian fissure.

the hemispheres aren't absolute. The two sides interact all the time and, depending on where the stroke has occurred, can sometimes make up for each other where small areas that have lost an ability to function are concerned. This brings us to the second good reason for having two hemispheres in the cerebral cortex. It provides an exquisite balance to our ability to perceive the world and respond accurately to it.

Overall, the two hemispheres do have characteristics that balance each other. The right hemisphere is the hemisphere that is usually involved with matters that affect our visual and spatial awareness. **Spatial awareness** is important for recognizing shapes, angles, and proportions. People with a stroke involving the right hemisphere may have trouble drawing simple images, even if they're given a model to copy. Not surprisingly, this is also the side of the brain that scientists have associated with use of the imagination, of making new connections out of old ideas—perhaps even "pulling them out of thin air." The right hemisphere can also affect our ability to recognize others, or even parts of our own body. Musical ability and a sense of pitch are also located in this hemisphere. (Sometimes a person who has trouble understanding spoken language after a stroke does better with understanding song. That may be because the right hemisphere hasn't been affected.)

John's family was upset. His wife, Jan, had just been to visit him in the hospital—and she had brought a surprise for him. It was a radio tuned to his favorite jazz station. He had shown no reaction to it at all. Jan was annoyed. She knew John loved jazz. He had always loved jazz. She decided to talk to their children.

In the days since John's stroke, his children had watched their father gradually regain his strength, though evidence of weakness on the left side of his body remained. What disturbed them more was the fact that he wasn't acting quite like himself, and he didn't act the same with some members of his family as he had before. His behaviors didn't add up to the father they knew and loved.

These things were enough to upset John's loved ones. But there was more. John just wasn't as concerned about his serious condition as his family thought he should be. In fact, he didn't seem to be concerned about anything at all. It was as though he couldn't admit that he had had a stroke, despite the fact that there he was, lying in a hospital bed. Talking with John could be a strange experience.

Trying to help him was frustrating, too. John consistently ignored efforts his family made to help rehabilitate his weak limbs. That didn't make their work any easier. The whole situation was beginning to make everyone feel a bit hurt, tired, and cross. Why wasn't John trying harder to help himself, seeing how hard they worked to help him?

Dr. James was John's attending physician. Jan decided to ask her if she could explain these troubling developments. Dr. James was reassuring. John's indifference to music, his lack of concern about his stroke, and his changed emotional reactions were all related, Dr. James said. They all involved behaviors controlled by the right hemisphere of the brain, where his rather large stroke had occurred. It was possible that some of these things might come back to some degree with time, but the family would have to wait and see.

John wasn't trying to be difficult, Dr. James emphasized. "Try not to get too frustrated with him, and concentrate instead on finding ways to compensate for his behavioral deficits," she said. "The nurses here can help you get started."

The left hemisphere rounds out the "interests" of the right hemisphere with complementary ones. The left side is considered the more "logical" side. Analytical thought and problem-solving come mainly from this area. Damage to the left hemisphere can result in noticeable problems with language and mathematical ability.

Scientists even find that complementary shadings of emotion color each hemisphere. While our emotions certainly aren't limited to certain sides of the brain, they do seem to have favorites. The right hemisphere is associated with negative emotions. A person with a stroke here might deny that anything bad has happened, even when it is pointed out to him. The left hemisphere seems to be more closely associated with positive emotions. An injury to this area could mean the person doesn't respond with appropriate enthusiasm to happy or positive events. She may be accused of being "sullen," but this is really not the case. She simply has lost the ability to express happy emotions.

The two hemispheres of the brain look almost identical, but even physically they have important differences. One hemisphere always has a slightly more developed, or **dominant,** area where written and spoken language is organized. In almost all of us, the left hemisphere is dominant for this big job. This is true for all right-handed people and most left-handed people. In some lefties, however, the area for language proficiency is larger in the right hemisphere instead. In some others, neither hemisphere is dominant.

Two Layers

The entire cerebrum is composed of two layers. The outermost layer is called the **cerebral cortex,** or **gray matter,** and it is here that man's unique ability to reason and make complicated move-

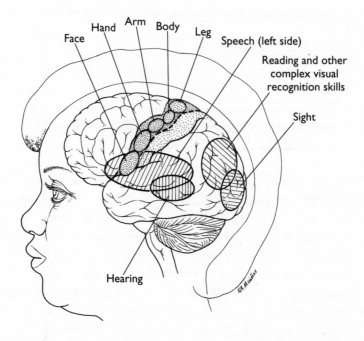

The motor cortex, which lies in front of the central fissure in each hemisphere, controls movements for the opposite side of the body.

ments lies. (The word *cortex* means "rind" or "rim.") Beneath the cerebral cortex lies the **white matter** of the brain. This enormous network of nerve fibers allows different parts of the cortex to communicate with each other. The cortex itself is deeply wrinkled. The "wrinkles" are actually folds that allow the cortex carpet to fold in on itself. That allows a greater amount of surface area to fit into the relatively small confines of the skull. And it allows a human being a great many more brain cells to think with than, say, a bird, which has a small, smooth cerebral cortex. If the cerebral cortex were taken out of the brain and allowed to expand to its full size when smooth, it would be about three times as large as it seems in the brain.

Three of the deepest folds are used as markers by neurologists to artificially divide the hemispheres into four distinct areas, or **lobes.** Each lobe of the cortex is responsible for different jobs. The **longitudinal sulcus** is the deep fissure that runs front to back down the center of the brain, separating the two cerebral hemispheres. A more shallow fissure runs along the side of each hemisphere, a little like a racing stripe. It is called the **Sylvian fissure.** Finally, the **central fissure** starts at the top of the brain, at the longitudinal sulcus, and drops down to meet the Sylvian fissure. The central fissure separates the frontal lobe from the parietal lobe. The tissue just in front of the central fissure is specialized for motor activities. The area just behind it is specialized for the input of touch and other body sensations.

The Frontal Lobe

The **frontal lobe,** naturally enough, lies in front of the central fissure. The frontal lobe itself can be divided into roughly three sections. The first, lying closest to the central fissure, is responsible for movements on the opposite side of the body. This area is known as the **motor cortex,** and it extends in a strip down from the top of the frontal lobe to the Sylvian fissure. In each hemisphere, the motor cortex is organized in the same way.

Neurons responsible for movement of the lower part of the body —including the toes and ankles—are found at the top of the strip. Neurons responsible for the movement of the middle parts of the body, such as the fingers, are found in the middle of the motor cortex. And those jobs involving the face, including the lips and tongue, are performed by neurons found at the bottom of this special part of the cortex. In addition, the amount of space each job is allotted depends on the complexity of the movement involved. Toes, which are limited in movement, get just a bit of space. But hands, which are capable of extremely delicate operations and are vitally important to human beings, get a lot.

Damage to the motor strip in one hemisphere can result in paralysis on the opposite side of the body. If the part of the strip that controls the lips, mouth, or tongue is involved, the person will have a certain difficulty pronouncing words, although his use of language will be correct and he will understand very well what is said. If the larger nearby areas of the frontal lobe are involved, the person will have difficulty getting the right word out. It can sound like a different word or no recognizable word at all.

Moving farther out toward the front of the brain, the motor movements become more complicated. A stroke involving this area could mean that the person has difficulty doing tasks that are sequential. He will repeat the first step over and over, unable to move on to the next step. In a classic test of this function, if such a person were given a piece of paper with boxes and circles on it and asked to cross out all the boxes and then all the circles, the person would get "stuck." He would be able only to cross out the boxes. Such a person would also find it hard to concentrate or plan ahead. For example, if the person went to the kitchen to make a sandwich, he might get out the bread and then forget what to do next. He wouldn't be able to complete complex tasks. He would not be able to plan motor activities and send signals to his muscles to do those things. He would also find it hard to comprehend a complicated idea.

Mark had brought Julia home a few weeks after her stroke, and they were still adjusting to some of her disabilities. The doctors said Julia's stroke had damaged the cortex in her frontal lobe, and she would have some weakness on her left side. Also, the doctors told Mark that the effects of the stroke would make Julia seem absentminded about some things. She also might not talk as much as before and might seem content to just sit and do nothing.

One evening, Julia decided she'd like a sandwich and headed for the kitchen to make it.

"I'll make you one, too, Mark," Julia said.

A little later, Mark went back to the kitchen to join Julia. He found her sitting at the kitchen table, looking upset. A loaf of bread lay on the table, but there were no sandwiches. Julia's stroke had made it difficult for her to complete sequential tasks, Mark remembered. His wife would get stuck on the first step and be unable to continue. Making a sandwich, he now reminded himself, took several steps from start to finish.

Reassuring Julia and offering to lend a hand, Mark started to help fix their snack. He first asked his wife to get the turkey. He then asked her to get the lettuce. He made a separate request for each item. Later, he thought, he would make a short list that Julia might follow the next time she wanted a sandwich. They chatted together for a while as they ate, and then Mark changed the subject.

"You know, dear, there are two great movies on TV to-night. One starts at eight, and the other starts at nine. I was thinking we could watch half of the first one and then try the second one and see how we like it. What do you think?"

Again, Julia looked frustrated and confused. Without realizing it, Mark had described a rather complicated plan for their evening. For someone who had had a stroke like Julia's, complicated ideas were just as difficult to follow as complicated actions. Mark caught himself, and posed the question again. "Shall we watch a movie tonight?"

"Yes, I'd like to," Julia said immediately.

"Later, could we watch a different movie?" he asked.

"Well, maybe," Julia said mischievously.

Finally, at the outermost portion of the frontal lobe lies the part of the brain where more abstract thinking occurs. Insight, initiative, and inhibition are generated from this area. Stroke survivors with damage in this area could become very uninhibited in their behaviors, speaking or acting inappropriately or impulsively. Or they might be hard to coax to talk, very inactive, or even extremely inert. Some might become apathetic and lose the initiative they once had to go to work or even do routine chores around the home. This condition is called **abulia,** which means "not enough behavior." It's as though the "spark plugs" of these people aren't firing properly to get them going. Although intellectually these people are the same as before, their loved ones will notice they have undergone a personality change.

The Parietal Lobe

The frontal lobe lies in front of the central fissure. Behind it lies the **parietal lobe,** at the back of the cerebral hemispheres. The frontal lobe deals mainly with motor activities—that is, movement—and sending signals. The parietal lobe is mainly concerned with sensory activities—that is, receiving information from the body that the brain can interpret.

A stroke involving the parietal lobe can impair tasks that require a sense of perspective, such as drawing. Told to copy a simple box

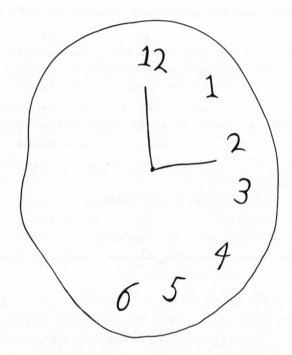

A stroke survivor with right-brain damage may have a spatial awareness problem called neglect. If so, he will completely ignore the left
side of his body as well as the left half of any objects placed in front of
him. If such a person is asked to copy a clock face, this is the type of
image he would draw. A person with neglect will also typically ignore
half a full plate of food or the people who visit him and sit on his left
side.

shape, someone with a stroke involving this area may only be able
to put down the parts in no particular order. As a result, the "box"
would look more like a jumble of sticks. This same person would
have trouble with maze puzzles. In walking around, he would have
a tendency to get lost easily. He may not recognize faces, either,
although he may recognize voices accurately. He can do this because hearing is concerned with a different part of the brain—the
temporal lobe.

We have seen that the frontal lobe has a specialized area next to
the central fissure that directs the movements of the body. In a
similar way, on the parietal side lies a specialized area called the
sensory cortex, which receives information from all parts of the

body. Other parts of the brain also receive information like this, but not as precisely as the sensory cortex. If a stroke occurs in this area, a person will still be able to feel sensations, but he won't be able to say what sensations they are or where he feels them. Scientists believe that the parietal lobes may be where knowledge is "put together" from the contributions of the rest of the cerebral hemisphere. Damage to the parietal lobes in the right hemisphere can result in a strange kind of disorder called **agnosia.** Stroke survivors with agnosia have perceptual disabilities. They may not be able to understand what they feel, see, or hear—despite the fact that touch, vision, and hearing are preserved.

Another perceptual disorder that may result from a stroke involving the parietal lobe is a condition known as **neglect.** People with neglect have a number of sensory deficits on the stroke-involved side of the body. The nature of their sensory deficit is to ignore everything on that side.

Shortly after Eric had a stroke, his best friend came by the hospital for a visit. Larry was surprised when Eric, who was sitting up in bed, ignored his greeting as he came through the door. Eric's wife, Martha, waved hello, though, and motioned Larry over to the right side of Eric's bed, where she was.

"We're just about to have lunch," Martha said.

"Larry! Glad to see you," Eric said suddenly, as Larry reached the bedside. Now Larry was thoroughly confused. Hadn't Eric already seen him come into the room?

"Eric's stroke has left him with some perceptual problems," Martha explained to Larry. "You have some trouble seeing things on your left, don't you, Eric?" she added, drawing her husband into the conversation.

"I guess," Eric responded vaguely.

The three friends chatted about other things for a while, until a nurse brought in Eric's lunch.

As Eric ate, Larry noticed his friend cleaned the right half of his plate, right to the middle, but didn't touch any food on the left side. Martha watched, too, and deftly turned the plate 180 degrees when Eric seemed finished. This put the rest of his lunch back on the right side of the plate. Eric immediately picked up his fork again and ate as though he had never been interrupted.

Larry left a short while later and promised to visit again soon. That evening, he called Martha at home and expressed some concern over Eric's behavior.

"Eric has a problem called 'neglect,' Larry," Martha said. "He consistently ignores whatever is happening to his left, which is why he didn't notice you at first when you came into his hospital room. That's why he eats just half of the food on his plate at a time. The doctor said that when Eric reads, he skips half the words on the page, too. He also ignores the left side of his body. He is so detached from it that yesterday he spotted his own arm and thought someone else was in bed with him!

"That sounds funny, but of course the underlying problem isn't. He could hurt himself if he doesn't develop an awareness of that side. His stroke affected the part of the brain that governs how the brain interprets sensations sent to it by the eyes, the fingertips, and other parts of the body on Eric's left side."

"What happens next?" Larry asked. "What can I do for you and Eric?"

"Eric and I have been working on exercises to help him learn to compensate for his left-side neglect. But the next time you visit, it would help if you could move over into his right-hand field of vision as soon as possible and sit over on his right side, too," Martha said.

"You know, neglect can be a very isolating condition," she added thoughtfully. "Eric didn't have great hearing or night vision as it was. Now, if he can't get strong input from his right side, I'm afraid he'll feel very left out of things. We all should keep his neglect in mind when we're with him. That would really help."

The Temporal Lobe

Below the Sylvian fissure lies the **temporal lobe.** This area is concerned mainly with hearing and memory, but it also is involved with auditory perception. The temporal lobes of each hemisphere have slightly different tasks. In most people, as we have discussed, the left hemisphere is dominant. The dominant hemisphere takes care of language and speech control, which also fall largely in the temporal lobe. Strokes on the dominant side in the temporal lobe can cause a condition known as **Wernicke's aphasia.** A person with this condition cannot make sense of what has been said to her and cannot monitor what she says herself. (Bear in mind that her ears and hearing are fine. The problem is back in the brain, where the impulses gathered by the ear are supposed to be organized into messages the brain can interpret.) This person will use the wrong words, or even made-up words, in sentences. Strangely, these sentences may accurately mimic the rhythms of speech. Upon closer investigation, however, they just don't make sense.

The temporal lobe is also where memories are believed to be stored. Usually, unless both lobes are affected by stroke, memory loss isn't permanent; the other hemisphere seems to compensate. Permanent memory loss is more likely if a stroke affects the **hippocampus,** part of the limbic system. This is fairly unusual, fortunately. Severe stroke damage to the hippocampus can mean that the brain loses its ability to create new memories. Long-term memory is unaffected—the person can recall everything that happened until just before her stroke. But she can't hang on to what she's just heard or seen. Within minutes it has slipped away.

The Occipital Lobe

Fourth and finally, the **occipital lobe** lies behind the temporal lobe, low in the cerebral hemisphere at the back of the head. Vision is so important to humans that it is accorded a lot of space in the cerebral cortex. Here is where all the complex individual signals collected by the eye are interpreted in a sensible way. A stroke involving one side of this area leaves a person blind to the opposite side in both eyes—even though the eyeballs are perfectly normal and able to function.

At age thirty-five Jack had always enjoyed perfect vision. That was until a recent stroke had left him partially blind in each eye. Now he was learning to compensate for the partial blindness so he could get back into a regular routine. But he was frequently frustrated.

"I could understand losing the vision in one eye and living with that," he told his doctor one day. "But with both eyes half-blind on the same side, I'm going crazy. I constantly run into things on the left side that I can't see. And it's hard to explain my situation to people."

Dr. Johnson listened sympathetically. "Your stroke occurred at the back of your head, on the right side. That is where the brain interprets the raw data related to the things you see on your left," she said. "In your case, the right occipital lobe, which interprets the left-hand side of your field of vision, was affected. That's why both eyes are partially blind on the same side, and not just one or the other eye."

She reminded Jack that with time, he would certainly adjust to his disability and find ways to compensate for it adequately. For instance, she suggested he scan rooms as a matter of course, moving his head from left to right, to get a more complete picture of the area around him. That could help prevent his being literally blindsided by objects on his left.

"How are you getting around town, Jack?" she asked. "You can't drive with this disability. It would be dangerous for you and others. How do you plan to get to work?"

"I've been thinking about that. There are a few people in my office who carpool from my part of town, so I may be able to join them if I chip in for gas. Some of my neighbors have offered to help me with some errands. Mainly, though, I'm investigating the bus system. It takes some getting used to, but it's worth it. It's really important to me to get around on my own steam."

Blood and the Brain

Making sure such a vast and complicated organ is adequately supplied with energy and oxygen is clearly quite a job. Now let's look closely at the blood vessel system that supplies the brain.

Blood reaches the brain from the heart through four major arterial systems. Two run up from the front of the neck. These are called the **carotid arteries.** These arteries mainly supply the frontal

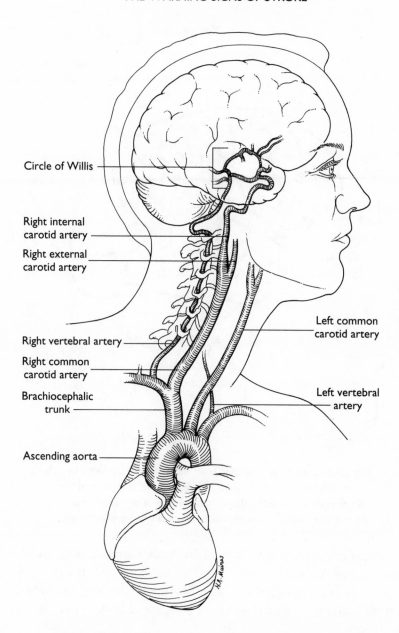

Circle of Willis

Right internal
carotid artery

Right external
carotid artery

Left common
carotid artery

Right vertebral artery

Right common
carotid artery

Brachiocephalic
trunk

Left vertebral
artery

Ascending aorta

Blood reaches the brain from the heart through four main arteries.
The two carotid arteries run up the front of the neck. They supply
the front and top of the brain with blood. Two vertebral arteries run
up the back of the neck. They supply the back and lower portions of
the brain with blood.

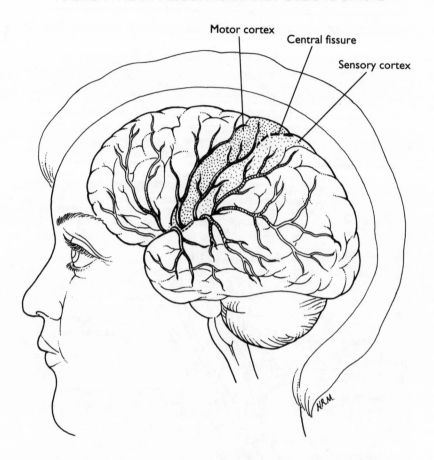

Motor cortex

Central fissure

Sensory cortex

Once inside the brain, the four main arteries from the neck branch and branch again, eventually supplying all parts of the brain with blood. This simplified illustration shows the way one of the larger branches, the middle cerebral artery, serves a part of one cerebral hemisphere.

and upper regions of the brain. Two smaller arteries are found at the back of the neck, where they become entwined in the spinal column before entering the brain. These are known as the **vertebral arteries,** and they mainly supply the back and bottom portions of the brain.

Once inside the skull, these four major arteries branch numerous times, first into a series of ever-smaller **cerebral arteries** and finally into a spidery web of tiny **capillaries.** In this way, every spot on the surface of the brain and within it is fully supplied with blood at all times.

A stroke occurs when one of the arteries carrying nutrients and oxygen to the brain either becomes clogged or ruptures. **Ischemic** strokes are caused by a lack of blood reaching the brain. They are the result of a clogged artery. **Hemorrhagic** strokes are caused by blood escaping from the vessels. They are the result of a ruptured blood vessel. During an ischemic stroke, the brain tissue and neurons that are fed by the clogged vessel start to die. The tissue at this point is considered **ischemic,** which translates literally to "withholding blood."

At this stage, which is often called a "stroke in progress," close to half of all stroke patients show a worsening of their symptoms. This period may last for the first few minutes or hours after the onset of the stroke. (Less commonly, stroke patients may worsen for other medical reasons as well.)

About one-fifth of all stroke patients show signs of a worsening condition after being hospitalized. Doctors will take careful notice of any evidence of the worsening of a patient's symptoms. Even the way symptoms present themselves can give doctors clues as to the type and location of the stroke.

"Worsening" falls into three categories. "Smooth worsening" indicates that the problem is gradually getting worse. "Steplike worsening" describes a neurologic deficit that increases rapidly one or more times, with periods of no change in between. "Fluctuating worsening" indicates that there has been at least one period of improvement preceding a worsening neurologic deficit.

During a stroke in progress, one of two things happens: The tissue either recovers or dies. The involved area may recover spontaneously if surrounding blood capillaries are able to compensate quickly enough for the missing blood flow. The larger the area of tissue involved, the more unlikely that this compensation will be complete, however. In some cases, the tissue may recover due to immediate medical treatment, but this option is relatively new and still in the early stage. We'll look at those developments more closely in Chapter Four.

If the involved tissue dies, the dead area is called an **infarct.** The nerve cells in this part of the brain will no longer be able to function, and therefore the part of the body they controlled won't be able to function normally, either. The dead cells will never be replaced by new ones. An infarct can result in a variety of outcomes, depending on which part of the brain is affected. Some people may have difficulty talking or walking; some may lose their memory. The symptoms may prove to be permanent or temporary.

Sometimes neighboring areas of the brain can compensate for the permanently damaged part. It may take time for the new connections to be forged. When that eventually happens, however, the associated tissue can "learn" some or all of the function that had been lost. The extent to which this is possible depends on things that vary from one person to the next. One is the area in which the infarct occurs. Another is its severity (how large it is). Sometimes this improvement occurs spontaneously. At other times it is helped along by rehabilitative exercises.

Recovery from a stroke depends on several elements: the amount and location of brain damage; the person's general health; his personality and emotional state; the support of family and friends; and the medical care he receives.

How Do Strokes Occur?

As we noted earlier, strokes occur when blood vessels either become clogged or rupture in the brain, killing affected tissue. Strokes caused by a lack of blood reaching the brain are called **ischemic,** while those caused by blood escaping from the vessels are called **hemorrhagic.**

The human cardiovascular system acts as the waterworks of the brain and other parts of the body. We know that water pipes can become clogged, depriving parts of the house of water. They can also break, releasing too much water into the wrong places. The same thing can happen to blood vessels in the brain. In the brain, blood vessels branch off to supply various "rooms" or parts of the brain.

From these two broad categories, ischemic and hemorrhagic, neurologists have defined several main types of stroke. Each type represents different causes, problems for the patient, effective treatments, and predicted outcomes. That's why making these distinctions is extremely important. We obviously wouldn't try to fix a leaking water pipe in the same way we would try to repair a blocked one; to do so would only make the original problem worse. The

---

COMMON TYPES OF STROKE

Thrombotic stroke. A thrombotic stroke is caused by a blood clot, or thrombus, that forms in an artery going to the brain. The clot blocks the passage of blood to a part of the brain. (This type of stroke accounts for about 60 percent of all strokes.)

Embolic stroke. An embolic stroke occurs when a brain artery is blocked by a clot that has formed elsewhere—usually in the heart or in the neck arteries—and been carried through the bloodstream to the brain. (This type of stroke accounts for about 20 percent of all strokes.)

Systemic hypoperfusion. In systemic hypoperfusion, blood flow to the brain is decreased because the heart fails to pump sufficiently. This happens, for example, after a cardiac arrest. These strokes are very different from the more common ischemic strokes because the damage is more diffuse and affects both sides of the brain. Some experts do not regard systemic hypoperfusion as a stroke.

Subarachnoid hemorrhage. A subarachnoid hemorrhage occurs when there is uncontrolled bleeding on the surface of the brain, in the area between the brain and the skull. This is usually caused by a rupture of an aneurysm, or bulge, in the wall of the artery. (This type of stroke accounts for about 10 percent of all strokes.)

Intracerebral hemorrhage. In this type of stroke, an artery deep within the brain ruptures and blood pressing into the brain tissue destroys it. (This type of stroke accounts for about 10 percent of all strokes.)

---

same truth applies to strokes, and for that reason doctors will determine as precisely as possible the type of stroke that has occurred. Fortunately, each of the two categories has its own general characteristics. Let's take a closer look at ischemic and hemorrhagic stroke and see what they are.

Ischemic Stroke

The most common type of stroke occurs when blood is prevented from delivering the necessary nutrients and oxygen to the brain because of blockages in the arteries. These **ischemic strokes** account for about three-quarters of all strokes. Typically, symptoms develop over a few minutes, though they may worsen over hours or days. Patients will show neurologic deficits such as paralysis on one side of the body or problems with speech and language.

The causes underlying this kind of stroke are numerous. Sometimes it takes a number of tests over a period of time before a doctor can make a final decision about which is most important. Patients with stroke are unlikely to have been completely healthy before their stroke, however. Most have a medical history that includes one or more risk factors for stroke. **Risk factors** for stroke are unfavorable health conditions and behaviors that can make a person more likely than others to have a stroke. Some important risk factors for stroke include **hypertension** (chronically high blood pressure), heart disease, smoking, and even previous stroke. The ischemic event itself is attributed to one of several conditions, which are discussed below.

Bob lit a cigarette just after eating his favorite carryout lunch—a big cheeseburger, french fries, a milk shake, and a slice of pie.

"I wish you wouldn't smoke so much," his wife sighed.

Bob shrugged. For years, friends, family, and doctors had been after him to stop smoking. But stopping was hard. Besides, he felt fine.

"Let's get back to the yard work, Bob," Nancy said, changing the subject.

Outside, Nancy and Bob worked together on the lawn. After about an hour Bob began to feel odd. His right side seemed to weaken, and it became difficult for him to continue raking. He called to his wife, but his speech came out all wrong.

Nancy got Bob inside. At first, they thought Bob was just tired. But after an hour, the weakness he felt had increased, and talking became more and more difficult.

"Look, Bob, I'd feel better if we could just go to the hospital and get you checked out," Nancy said. "I'll drive."

Shortly after Bob was seen in the emergency room, Dr. Harper approached Nancy.

"You did the right thing in bringing your husband here," Dr.

Harper said gently. "Our tests confirm that he's had a minor embolic stroke." The doctor went on to explain that he needed to admit Bob to the hospital for treatment. He also assured Nancy that Bob had a good chance for a full recovery.

When Bob was ready to go home from the hospital, Dr. Harper went over the risk factors for stroke and gave him diet and exercise information along with a brochure on stopping smoking.

"Bob, you have recovered well from your stroke. But there are some things you can do to help prevent another stroke."

Bob went home and sat down with Nancy.

"Nancy, I know I can give up cheeseburgers and other fatty foods. Giving up smoking will be harder. But others have done it, and so can I."

"I know you can," Nancy assured him.

"Exercise?" he asked. "Now there's a problem. Dr. Harper said I don't have to jog. But he does want me to exercise more."

"Let's go for a walk and talk about it," Nancy suggested.

Bob reached for his cigarettes. Much to Nancy's surprise, he threw them into the trash. He put his arm around her shoulder. "Let's go," he said. "You know, we used to love to ride bikes when we were younger. Maybe we should get our bikes out and tune them up a bit."

Thrombotic Stroke

Thrombotic stroke occurs when a cerebral artery is blocked off by a clot that forms along the vessel wall, preventing the passage of blood. A thrombosis can also develop in any of the four neck arteries that carry blood from the heart to the brain.

A thrombosis doesn't occur in healthy arteries. Usually it is the result of a disorder called **atherosclerosis,** sometimes called hardening of the arteries, which is common in adults. The condition gets started when the inner lining of the blood vessels becomes injured. This injury may be caused by normal wear and tear of substances in the bloodstream constantly brushing past and by the pounding of high blood pressure. Fats—cholesterol—from the blood accumulate along the vessel walls in fatty streaks. A rough

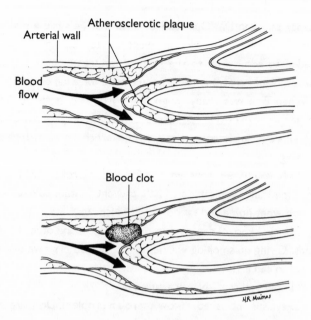

Atherosclerosis is an abnormal condition of the arteries in which a thick, rough deposit forms on the inner wall of the arteries and gradually narrows the passageway so that blood flow is slowed.

If an artery has been damaged by atherosclerosis, it can develop roughened places that stick out into the bloodstream. Blood clots are likely to form around those places. When a blood clot is large enough to block blood from passing, a thrombotic infarction occurs, which is illustrated here.

deposit called **plaque** develops, made out of the fats, or **lipids,** and other substances in the blood that catch on the rough spots. The part of the vessel through which blood can pass becomes smaller and smaller as this process continues. This kind of change in the artery is called **stenosis.** Blood clots may form over the roughened places in the artery, too. These clots, or thromboses, may block the vessel completely (an occlusion), causing a thrombotic stroke. Alternatively, they may break away and be carried downstream, where they cause an embolic stroke.

Embolic Stroke

An **embolus** is a wandering clot or other undissolved material that has been carried through the bloodstream until it hits an artery too small to pass through, blocking it and causing an infarction, or

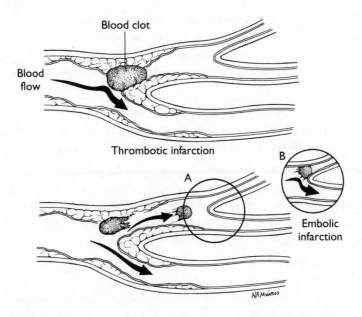

Sometimes a smaller blood clot breaks off from a larger one (A) and is carried elsewhere in the bloodstream. It might come from a neck artery or a diseased heart. This wandering blood clot is called an embolus. It stops when it reaches an artery through which it cannot pass (B), blocking the blood behind it from passing as well. An embolic infarction results.

stroke. Often an embolus is a piece of a blood clot that has broken away from a diseased artery wall in the neck or from the inside wall of a diseased, poorly functioning heart. This is one reason doctors carefully examine a patient's heart history and function when assessing stroke damage. Emboli can occur throughout the body. They are called brain emboli when they get stuck in an artery within the head and cause a stroke. Emboli are estimated to account for about 20 percent of all strokes.

Lacunes

These small brain infarcts are caused by blockage of small penetrating arteries deep in the substance of the brain. They are called **lacunes** because of the tiny cavities or "lakes" they leave behind when the infarcted brain tissue withers away. No final agreement on their cause or causes has been reached. Some researchers believe lacunes result from a degenerative process caused by chronic high blood pressure that thickens artery walls until blood can no longer pass. Other evidence suggests that these infarcts can be caused by many conditions, including other local arterial diseases and emboli. Lacunes account for about 25 percent of all ischemic strokes.

Systemic Hypoperfusion (Low Blood Flow)

In some cases, an ischemic stroke results from a situation quite different from the blood and vessel problems just described. Sometimes strokes occur because of a circulatory failure caused by the heart itself. The heart's pumping action may fail and result in an inadequate output of blood. The blood pressure level is too low to pump the blood throughout the circulatory system, and too little blood may reach the brain. The result is circulatory failure, or systemic hypoperfusion.

Hypoperfusion affects the brain quite differently from the way thrombotic, embolic, or lacunar conditions do. Under those conditions, an infarct is created at the center of the area supplied by the artery. Circulation from surrounding arteries continues strongly, limiting the brain damage to a great extent. But in the case of hypoperfusion, the outermost regions of the brain on both sides or the entire brain is affected instead. These regions aren't serviced by any one artery but depend on a smaller blood supply from several neighboring arteries. When hypoperfusion occurs, all of these arteries are compromised at the same time. Blood simply can't reach the outermost areas it's supposed to supply with oxygen and nutrients. It's as if the water pressure suddenly drops as you are watering the lawn: You can still water the area around your feet, but you find it impossible to reach the outer edges of the grass with the spray. If the water pressure drops low enough, no water comes out of the hose at all. This is when cardiac arrest occurs. All circulation to the brain ceases, and infarction of the entire brain occurs.

Hemorrhagic Stroke

Not all strokes are caused by conditions that prevent blood from reaching the brain. Fifteen to 20 percent are caused by the rupture of a blood vessel in or around the brain. These hemorrhagic strokes fall into two categories: **subarachnoid hemorrhage** and **intracerebral hemorrhage.** In either case, some part of the brain is deprived of the energy normally supplied by blood in the artery involved,

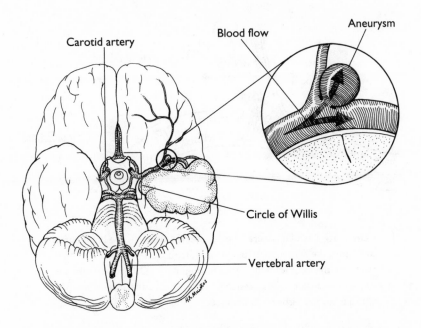

Carotid artery

Blood flow

Aneurysm

Circle of Willis

Vertebral artery

Aneurysms like the one illustrated above indicate weak spots in the artery wall. These weak spots were present at birth. Aneurysms don't usually develop, however, until adolescence or, more often, adulthood, when the weak spots balloon out and fill with blood. They are often associated with high blood pressure. When aneurysms burst, they cause subarachnoid or intracerebral hemorrhage.

which kills the affected tissue. In addition, blood from the ruptured artery flows into unwelcome areas, displacing the brain tissue there and interfering with its function. Hemorrhagic strokes are usually more severe than ischemic strokes.

A variety of conditions contribute to or cause hemorrhage. Some of them, such as aneurysms, can't be controlled. **Aneurysms** are weak spots in the blood vessel wall. Not everyone has aneurysms, but those who do are generally born with defects in arteries that produce them. Aneurysms are believed to be congenital. The word *aneurysm* comes from the Greek for "widening." Aneurysms can generate over time, ballooning in size and stretching an already thin vessel wall even thinner. Eventually the blood vessel may rupture or burst, like a balloon inflated beyond its limits. High blood pressure can contribute to this process.

High blood pressure, especially when not controlled, is also inde-

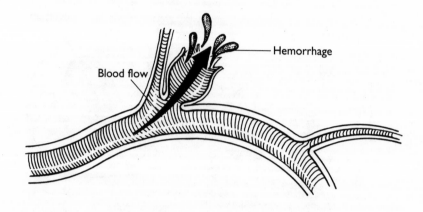

Blood flow

Hemorrhage

Hemorrhagic stroke occurs when a diseased artery in the brain bursts and floods the surrounding tissue with blood. Some parts of the brain can't get the oxygen and nutrients they need. Other parts are destroyed because of compression—clotted blood that collects in part of the brain and displaces brain tissue.

dependently associated with brain hemorrhage. This is true whether or not aneurysms are present. Drug abuse, too, is increasingly associated with brain hemorrhage in younger people, especially the use of cocaine, amphetamines, and alcohol.

A person's reaction to the onset of a hemorrhagic stroke can vary according to the size and location of the bleeding into the brain. The escape of blood into the skull increases pressure within the closed space, causing a severe headache. Other symptoms of brain hemorrhage include decreased alertness and vomiting.

Subarachnoid Hemorrhage

The brain sits snugly within the skull, the bony fortress that protects it. The interior of the skull is just slightly larger than the brain itself. To protect the brain, layers of membranes and a cushion of **cerebrospinal fluid** are sandwiched between the soft brain and the hard skull. Uncontrolled bleeding into this area is called a **subarachnoid hemorrhage (SAH).**

The most common cause of SAH is a ruptured aneurysm, often in conjunction with high blood pressure. This combination is present in more than half of people with SAH due to ruptured aneurysms. It may take years for aneurysms to wear out and rupture, which may partially explain why the typical person with SAH is between forty and sixty years old.

Aneurysms are usually found at the branching points of arteries —places of high turbulence and stress for the blood vessel. If an aneurysm breaks, blood escapes into the cerebrospinal fluid around the brain. Generally speaking, the larger the aneurysm, the more likely it is to rupture. Larger aneurysms, not surprisingly, also cause bigger, more damaging hemorrhages.

Subarachnoid hemorrhages can also result from other problems, such as the rupture of an **arteriovenous malformation (AVM).** AVMs, like aneurysms, are congenital. They are made up of many thin-walled vessels that can burst and allow blood to leak into the brain substance, destroying or displacing it. These occur most commonly on the surface of the brain. Subarachnoid hemorrhages can also be caused by bleeding from an injury due to a blow to the head. The escape of blood from within the brain into the subarachnoid space can also be called a subarachnoid hemorrhage.

Most subarachnoid hemorrhages are the result of arterial problems. Blood flowing through the arteries comes directly from the heart. It is forced quickly on its way by the heart's pumping action. Even when there is a break in a vessel, that strong pumping action continues, forcefully pushing blood through the rupture and into the parts of the brain where it shouldn't go. The effect is dramatic, with an abrupt onset of symptoms.

Other hemorrhages are the result of venous or capillary problems. A rupture of a vein, which returns blood to the lungs to pick up more oxygen, usually causes damage more gradually. Farther removed from the heart's pumping action, blood flowing through the veins is under less forceful pressure. Thus leaks on this side of the vascular system are slower and may cause symptoms that appear over a period of time. AVM bleeding is usually capillary or venous.

A person experiencing an SAH may develop an extremely severe headache within seconds, accompanied by pain and stiffness in the neck. He may describe this headache as "the worst in my life." Often, too, the person's consciousness level will change noticeably —he may exhibit anything from confusion to drowsiness to total unresponsiveness, or coma. Other general symptoms include dizziness and double vision. The hemorrhage increases pressure around the brain rather than affecting the brain itself, so people don't usually show the kind of specific symptoms most often associated with stroke, such as paralysis of a limb.

Paula, a middle-aged African American, was a principal at a middle school. She had returned to her office from a teachers' meeting early one morning when she was struck by a sudden, blinding headache that made her stagger. Sure, those breakfast meetings were always grueling, she thought, but they've never caused a headache this terrible. Not only was it the worst she could remember, but it gave her a painful, stiff neck as well. She felt nauseated and suddenly vomited in the wastepaper basket.

For a brief moment she wondered if her blood pressure had gone through the roof again. She took her medication—usually. Maybe she was having some kind of reaction to the pills. But in another moment that thought was replaced with the urge just to sit down. She had never felt this bad before—dizzy, weak, and drowsy.

When Ellen, her secretary, came in a moment later, she found Paula slumped in her chair. The principal hardly responded to her secretary's alarmed questions.

Ellen called for an ambulance immediately. At the hospital a short while later, Paula was diagnosed as having a subarachnoid hemorrhage. An aneurysm on the surface of the brain had ruptured, spilling blood into the fluid around the brain.

Intracerebral Hemorrhage

Intracerebral hemorrhage (ICH) is caused by bleeding into the tissue deep within the brain. Hypertension, chronically high blood pressure, has been pegged as the main culprit behind this type of stroke. The condition causes degenerative changes in the small arteries that can eventually cause the vessel to burst. There has been a sharp decline recently in the number of intracerebral hemorrhages in this country. A primary reason for this is increased public awareness of the danger of hypertension and the importance of controlling it.

Unfortunately, ICH due to causes other than hypertension is increasing. More cases are being traced to recreational drug use, complications from anticoagulant therapy (blood-thinning treatment), aneurysms, AVMs, brain tumors, and other problems.

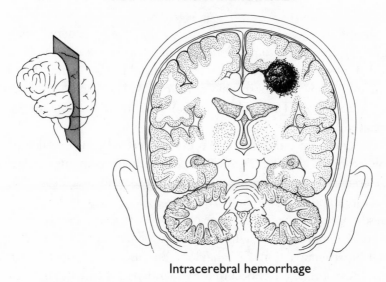

Intracerebral hemorrhage

Blood that escapes from a blood vessel and collects in the substance of the brain as illustrated here is called an intracerebral hemorrhage. The escaped blood collects and presses heavily on the brain, destroying brain tissue in the affected area.

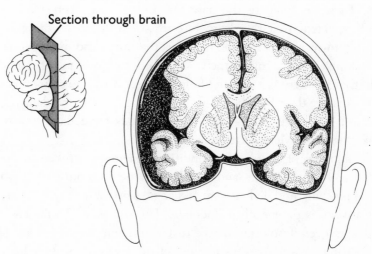

Section through brain

Subarachnoid hemorrhage

Bleeding from a ruptured vessel on the surface of the brain is called a subarachnoid hemorrhage, illustrated above. Bleeding here seeps into the limited space between the brain and skull. Increased pressure in the head can result.

35

Symptoms caused by ICH fall into two categories: **general symptoms** and **focal symptoms.** General symptoms are caused by uncontrolled bleeding, regardless of its location in the brain. Focal symptoms show up in specific parts of the body and vary from person to person. They indicate where in the brain the hemorrhage occurred.

General symptoms reflect the pressure exerted by the extra blood volume inside the skull, which forces the brain contents to shift and compress to compensate. General symptoms include headache, vomiting, and a change in alertness level. Very large hemorrhages cause stupor or coma; the chance of recovery in these cases is small.

Focal symptoms are a little different. Each part of the brain controls specific actions or behaviors. Because of this, doctors can tell where a stroke has occurred by identifying a patient's specific problem, or focal symptom. Paralysis of a limb and blindness in one eye are examples of focal symptoms.

The Warning Signs of Stroke

When we compare the data for strokes at a given age, it's apparent that the death rate for stroke has been dropping steadily in recent years. One reason is that more and more people are taking an active role in their own health care. It's quite possible that they're learning to do the following: eat better; exercise regularly; manage their high blood pressure, heart disease, and diabetes; and stop—or never start—smoking. We'll talk more about how to make these lifestyle changes in later chapters.

Sometimes, of course, the conditions leading to stroke can develop anyway. Smokers and people with heart conditions, high blood pressure, and diabetes are at a greater risk of having a stroke, but anyone is potentially vulnerable. The risk of stroke increases with age, even if no other risk factors are present.

Researchers are investigating a number of ways to stop or limit the effects of stroke medically. But doctors already agree that the sooner they can get to a person who is having a stroke, the better their chances of limiting the amount of brain damage and disability that may occur. And stopping a stroke before it starts—practicing preventive medicine—is best of all.

Doctors will sometimes catch the signs of an impending stroke when they see a patient for another reason. But each person can learn to look for the warning signals in himself—and then see a doctor as soon as possible. **A stroke demands immediate emergency medical care.**

The warning signs of stroke are the same whether you've already had a stroke or never have had one before. The warning signs can come intermittently and leave no lasting effect. These signs are called **transient ischemic attacks,** or **TIAs**. They indicate that the blood supply is being briefly disrupted. A total blockage may occur in the next few hours or days if treatment is not started.

Your body can warn you of a stroke before it happens. **Know the following warning signs. See a doctor promptly if you experience one or more of them.** Your body may be trying to tell you something. If you're at known risk for stroke, make sure your family and friends know these warning signs as well. That way, they can take quick action if you're incapacitated or unable to recognize your own symptoms.

THE WARNING SIGNS OF A STROKE

• Sudden weakness or numbness of the face, arm, or leg on one side of the body

• Sudden dimness or loss of vision, particularly in one eye

• Loss of speech, or trouble talking or understanding speech

• Sudden, severe headaches with no apparent cause

• Unexplained dizziness, unsteadiness, or sudden falls, especially along with any of the previous symptoms

---

Transient Ischemic Attacks— An Important Signal

Many people experience an important harbinger of a major stroke called a transient ischemic attack (TIA), or "temporary stroke." About 20 to 40 percent of strokes are preceded by

TIAs. They occur days, weeks, or months before a major stroke. TIAs are identified by a combination of the symptoms above.

TIAs typically come on rapidly and last five to fifteen minutes. Some people have just one episode; others experience a cluster of TIAs over a few days or weeks. Then the symptoms disappear as swiftly as they appeared. None of the symptoms—numbness, blindness, paralysis, weakness—last. The person may feel completely normal.

But don't be fooled. Everything is far from normal. TIAs are extremely important warning signs for stroke and should never be ignored. In fact, people who have had TIAs are almost ten times more likely to have a stroke soon thereafter than people of the same age and sex who haven't had a TIA.

Small emboli are believed to be the most common cause of TIAs. They are carried through the blood until they lodge in a small artery. They may be dissolved by substances in the blood before any lasting brain damage is done. Because there is no residual evidence left after the episode, however, it's impossible to know exactly what causes TIAs. It may be a combination of factors. TIAs are much more closely associated with subsequent ischemic rather than hemorrhagic strokes.

"I feel kind of silly coming to see you, doctor," Tom said when his doctor entered the examining room. "But something happened yesterday that worried me, so here I am."

Dr. Polk urged Tom to describe the incident.

"Well, what happened didn't hurt and it didn't last long," Tom began. Now he almost wondered if it had happened at all. But his wife agreed that it had, so here he was. "It was strange. One minute I was making the bed, and the next I was stopped cold and had to sit down."

"What do you mean by 'stopped cold'?" Dr. Polk asked.

"I became very weak—but only on one side of my body. The right, I think. The room got dark suddenly. I couldn't see very well. And when I tried to call my wife into the room, I just couldn't make my mouth work—everything came out garbled," Tom remembered. "I felt awkward—clumsy."

"These symptoms all came on rapidly?" Dr. Polk asked.

"Yes, and they stopped just as quickly, too. In about two minutes or so, the whole episode was over, and I felt fine, absolutely fine. But it shook me up. It didn't seem right."

Tom was right about that. What he described, the doctor knew, were symptoms of a classic TIA, or "mini-stroke." Dr. Polk admitted Tom to the hospital and ordered several tests. Those tests revealed that a problem with the left carotid artery had caused Tom's TIA. Dr. Polk assured Tom that the condition could be treated with surgery to the artery.

In the final analysis, warning signs or TIAs show that something is wrong, but they do not show exactly what is amiss. They are generally painless, which makes them easy to ignore—especially since they go away, anywhere from a few seconds to a few hours later. Although some TIAs occasionally last for several hours, it's uncommon for them to last more than thirty minutes. But don't ever ignore warning signs or TIAs! Seeing your doctor promptly is critical after experiencing any warning signs. She will determine whether a stroke has occurred or whether some other medical problem with similar symptoms (such as migraine or heart trouble) is mimicking a stroke.

The bottom line is: Know the warning signs of stroke. That knowledge can be as important to a personal stroke prevention program as following a sensible diet and keeping high blood pressure under control. Don't ignore the signs. Getting prompt medical attention is really up to you. It can mean the difference between a severely disabling stroke, a milder one, or none at all. It can even mean the difference between life and death.

Now we have an idea of how stroke happens. Next, let's take a look at who is likely to have a stroke and what can be done to control or eliminate that risk.

2
What Causes Stroke and Who Gets One?

We've started our discussion about stroke by looking at what happens inside the brain when a stroke occurs. But that is really the climax of a story that started in most cases many years before. A stroke happens most often because of damage to vessels that prevents them from supplying a certain part of the brain with blood. But what causes that initial damage?

The answer is a complex one, and it is different for every person. But today doctors know better than ever before what some of the most important risk factors for stroke are. They also know what can be done to eliminate them or make their effects less severe. And they are learning more all the time.

The fact is, the death rate from stroke has fallen over 50 percent in the United States since 1972. Much of the credit for this wonderful news has been attributed to one very important development. That is the public's better understanding and management of the risk factors that contribute to cerebrovascular disease over time. Most important among these are hypertension (high blood pressure) and atherosclerosis (a vessel disease). Both conditions will be discussed more fully in this chapter.

But far too many people still experience deadly or debilitating strokes each year. People who have high blood pressure and hardening of the arteries and smoke cigarettes are at particular risk of stroke. Those who have increased cholesterol levels, don't exercise, or are overweight may also be at high risk. The earlier in life that you begin to control or eliminate these factors, the better. Stroke prevention should be everyone's goal. The brain is vulnerable to the slightest damage. For this reason doctors believe that prevention will remain the key to reducing death and disability from stroke in the future. They believe prevention will be even more important than improvements in medical and surgical treatments called for after a stroke has occurred.

Practicing prevention, of course, depends on learning what the risk factors are for stroke in the first place. Let's get started. Chapter Eight will discuss prevention strategies in more detail.

Identifying Risk Factors

Identifying personal risk factors for stroke can be a little like sorting out clues in a good detective novel. To solve the mystery, one has to collect all the clues and put them together in a way that makes sense. Some clues carry more weight than others, and some are important only in association with other facts. Some clues are a product of the environment in which the story takes place. Risk factors often intertwine and affect each other. You may want to get your doctor's help in uncovering your own risk factors. The reward is well worth the effort. Identifying and evaluating risk factors opens the door to eliminating them or modifying their effects.

It's important to point out right away that risk factors are not absolutes. If you have one risk factor or a combination of them, it doesn't automatically mean you'll have a stroke. It *does* mean that you are more likely to have a stroke than if you didn't have those risk factors. How much more likely depends on which risk factors you have and how many. Even people without any identifiable risk factors, however, can still have a stroke, though their chances are smaller.

At age forty, Clay was the regional sales manager of a large Midwestern corporation. He was under constant pressure to meet his company's current goals and to inspire others to do the same.

For years Clay had met with clients and colleagues almost daily over lunch, dinner, drinks, and for other occasions. This lifestyle had taken its toll on him. Clay smoked and drank heavily, calling it the price of doing business in a social setting. As he liked to tell his colleagues, he "worked hard and partied hard."

A big man, he ate with gusto, too. He favored steakhouses with a cocktail bar when he entertained clients. He chose fast food drive-throughs for quick lunches when he was on his own. Clay was about thirty pounds overweight. Not only did he have a rich diet, but he just never seemed to find the time to get any real exercise.

"My business schedule during the week is far too hectic and uncertain for that," he would tell his wife. "By the weekend I'm too tired, and sick of going out, besides. I'd rather catch up on a little TV and relax with a beer in my own home."

One Saturday, Clay was doing just that when his face went numb and he seemed to lose vision to one side. The sportscaster on the TV program he was watching stopped making sense, too. Clay didn't know what to do next. He sat there for a little while and tried to think. Within fifteen minutes the episode passed and his symptoms disappeared.

Still, Clay was disturbed, especially by the strange, brief unintelligibility of that TV sportscaster. When he told his wife about it, she strongly urged him to see a doctor. When Clay did go to see Dr. Story, she told him he had had a TIA and needed a full evaluation. Clay had had a strong warning of a possible impending major stroke.

Clay was admitted to the hospital. The evaluation showed normal heart functioning. However, a plaque in his carotid artery had broken loose and temporarily blocked a blood vessel to his eye and brain. Dr. Story placed Clay on ticlopidine, a drug that affects platelet function in order to prevent further emboli. She also talked to him about preventive measures.

"Clay, we've talked about your health habits before," Dr. Story said. "Now we must act. In addition to being overweight, you've developed high blood pressure. You smoke, you drink too much, and you don't exercise. Together these factors are associated with a much higher than average risk of stroke, not to mention heart disease. This TIA was just your body's warning that something more serious is brewing. If you don't address your risks now, you are very likely to have a full-blown stroke. Believe me."

Clay followed Dr. Story's orders. He took his ticlopidine regularly as prescribed. He also quit smoking and joined a company support group of ex-smokers. When he felt tempted to light up because he was tense or in a social setting, he chewed gum instead.

Next, Dr. Story put Clay on a diet to help him lose weight safely and bring down his high blood pressure. Clay learned to keep track of his blood pressure. The diet cut out much of the fat and salt that Clay had grown accustomed to. He learned to replace most of his usual rich fare with leaner meats and more grains, pastas, vegetables, and fruits. He and his wife learned to prepare foods simply, with a minimum of fats and oils.

Clay still was reluctant to commit to a vigorous, regular exercise program. He did make a few small compromises. He started to walk around the neighborhood after dinner several nights a week with his wife and kids. This new routine gave them an added bonus—a quiet opportunity to talk. At work, Clay started parking at the end of the lot instead of next to the entrance. This gave him a short distance to walk each morning and evening. He also began to walk between office floors instead of taking the elevator. "Taking the stairs actually wakes me up a little, instead of making me tired," Clay observed with surprise to a colleague.

Gradually, Clay incorporated all these changes into his daily routine. He found new restaurants offering lighter cuisine. One was a trendy Japanese place that was a big hit with clients. He drank less. When he didn't have a lunch date scheduled, he brought his own lunch with fresh, lean foods from home.

Today, Clay looks better and feels better than he did a year ago. He credits that frightening TIA for the changes he made. Dr. Story is pleased with Clay's progress. She says Clay's new behaviors have indeed reduced his stroke risk.

As we've suggested, all risk factors for stroke aren't created equal. They fall into three broad categories: those that can't be changed; those that can be changed by medical treatment; and those that can be changed by lifestyle adjustment.

Risk factors that can't be changed include your age, sex, and race. They also include a history of a prior stroke and, at the present time, the presence of diabetes mellitus.

Risk factors that can be changed by medical treatment and/or lifestyle changes include high blood pressure, heart disease, and transient ischemic attacks (TIAs).

Several risk factors can be changed by lifestyle adjustments. A primary risk factor in this category is smoking. There are also several secondary risk factors in this category. They include cholesterol levels in the blood, obesity, exercise habits, and excessive alcohol intake. Secondary risk factors indirectly affect the risk of stroke by increasing the risk of heart disease, which itself is a primary risk factor for stroke. Smoking and excessive alcohol intake damage cerebral vessels as well.

At least some of these risk factors apply to most Americans to some degree. Let's take a closer look at them now.

What's My Risk?

The bad news is that almost all of us have some risk of having a stroke at some time in our lives. One reason is that we all grow a little older every day. Age is an important risk factor for stroke (as we'll see in a minute). However, there is good news, too: Almost everyone can take significant steps to reduce that personal risk.

A good place to start is with regular medical checkups. All in all, they are one of the best protections against stroke. By evaluating your medical history and examining you, your doctor can uncover conditions that may predispose you to stroke. She can then help you to get them under control immediately.

Timeliness is very important. The earlier preventive treatment can begin, the more effective it will be.

HOW TO REDUCE YOUR RISK OF STROKE

Have your blood pressure checked once a year. High blood pressure is the major risk factor for stroke.

Don't smoke cigarettes. Smoking increases the risk of heart attack and stroke. Heart disease itself is a risk factor for stroke.

Eat nutritious foods in moderate amounts. Eat a well-balanced diet that's low in cholesterol and saturated fats and moderate in sodium (salt). Fatty foods contribute to atherosclerosis, which itself is a major contributor to stroke.

Have regular medical checkups. Many risk factors call for medical supervision. These include high blood pressure, elevated cholesterol, excess weight, lack of exercise, and cigarette smoking. Getting these under control can help prevent a heart attack or stroke.

Know the warning signs. Prompt medical attention to the following symptoms could prevent a fatal or disabling stroke from occurring:
- Sudden weakness or numbness of the face, arm, or leg on one side of the body
- Sudden dimness or loss of vision, particularly in one eye
- Loss of speech, or trouble talking or understanding speech
- Sudden, severe headaches with no apparent cause
- Unexplained dizziness, unsteadiness, or sudden falls, especially along with any of the previous symptoms

---

Some Risk Factors We Have to Live With

Unfortunately, changing daily habits or taking advantage of medical treatment won't get rid of all of the risk factors for stroke. There are some we just have to live with. Still, they are important to recognize because their presence tends to increase the seriousness of other risk factors that can be controlled.

Age

Aging by itself doesn't cause stroke, but it is a primary risk factor for the disease. No matter who you are, your risk of having a stroke increases steadily with age. Almost three-quarters of all stroke cases in a given year affect people who are aged sixty-five years or older. And that risk more than doubles with each decade after sixty-five.

Older age as a risk factor may represent the long-term conse-quences of various conditions and behaviors on the body's cerebro-vascular system. These include high blood pressure, atherosclerosis, smoking, and other behaviors. Atherosclerosis, a disease of the arteries, is present to some degree in almost everyone over the age of forty, for example. High blood pressure, too, tends to increase with age for unknown reasons and should be aggressively treated. In the past, high blood pressure was considered a "natural" conse-quence of aging and was often overlooked for treatment except in the most extreme cases.

It's possible that as more people begin earlier to practice habits that keep these and other risk factors under control, the relative importance of age as a risk factor may decline. But for now and for the near future, being older than sixty-five years of age remains a significant risk for stroke. And as the American population ages, more people will be at risk for stroke.

Sex

At any particular age, men are more likely to have a stroke than women. Women mustn't rest easy, however. Even though men are at greater risk for stroke, stroke is still a major killer of women. That is because women tend to outlive men into the older age groups in which most strokes occur.

In 1989, the last year for which figures are available, women accounted for more than 60 percent of the 145,551 stroke deaths in the United States. Younger women who smoke and also take oral contraceptives are at a significantly high risk for stroke. This special case is discussed later in this chapter with other risks that can be controlled.

Family History

Stroke is a complex affliction, with multiple risk factors. Evidence is developing to indicate that some of these risk factors may be genetic. A susceptibility to hypertension, for example, is now thought to have a genetic component. Studies have shown that if neither parent is hypertensive, their offspring have scant chance of developing the disease. But if one parent has high blood pressure, their children have a one-in-five chance of developing the condition. And if both parents have high blood pressure, one in three of their children will probably also be hypertensive.

Other risk factors that can drop out of the family tree include a susceptibility to diabetes mellitus and atherosclerosis. Special conditions may be required before these problems develop, however. Obesity may contribute to the development of diabetes. Smoking and a poor diet may contribute to the development of atherosclerosis. These tendencies may surface as the result of an individual's unique genetic makeup. Or it may be that a genetic predisposition to stroke can be suppressed or delayed from developing if these triggers are controlled. Controlling these factors is a good idea in any case because doing so will improve your general health.

From these findings it is reasonable to conclude that a family history of stroke is also a strong risk factor for the illness. If others in your family background have experienced stroke, diabetes, hypertension, or heart disease, be sure to discuss it with your doctor.

Race

By the year 2000, minorities are expected to make up fully one-quarter of the United States population. Studies are beginning to show that some variations do exist between races in the types and underlying causes of strokes they get. As knowledge in these areas increases, better treatment will result for everyone at risk of stroke.

African Americans are in much greater danger of having a stroke than are other minority groups or Caucasians. Blacks are fully 60 percent more likely than whites to have a stroke.

Variations in cause of stroke and stroke type are emerging in other areas as well. Obese African Americans, for example, especially women, have been shown to have very high risk of heart failure. They also have very high risk of developing high blood pressure, diabetes, and stroke. But obese Native Americans and Hispanics in the Southwest don't seem to develop either high blood pressure or stroke as often as blacks. However, they do seem to be more susceptible to diabetes than African Americans are.

Genetic factors are thought to explain some of the differences in these and other examples, but environment may be a factor as well. The varying risks of high blood pressure discussed in the preceding paragraph, for example, may involve many other factors. Differences in dietary habits, the type of obesity, how quickly the weight is gained, and the age at which one becomes obese may also be important to the story.

Scientists involved in one recent preliminary study have found differences in the distribution of stroke risk factors among the three ethnic groups it researched. For minority patients who had a brain infarction, high blood pressure was slightly more prevalent in blacks and Hispanics than whites. Researchers also found that diabetes is more of a risk factor for stroke for Hispanics than for whites or blacks. This study also found that individual heart problems, including angina, myocardial infarction (heart attack), and atrial fibrillation (in which a part of the heart beats out of its normal rhythm) did not significantly differ among the three groups. However, whites who had strokes were found to be more likely to have a combination of these cardiac problems than any other group, while Hispanics were the least likely. In other studies, Asians, like African Americans, have also shown a stronger tendency for developing high blood pressure than whites. If the findings hold up under further study, it could mean more tailored prevention treatment and stroke care will be indicated for minorities.

The evidence is mounting that differences do exist in the way risk factors are distributed among the different ethnic groups. A person's race, then, may be a marker that indicates the degree of importance a particular risk factor has on one's total risk profile. It suggests that one's background may indicate a need for certain risk factors to be treated more aggressively.

Stroke mortality rates have declined steadily since 1962, and the decline has been most marked among African Americans. But blacks are still more likely than any other group in this country to have a stroke. Black women are around 80 percent more likely to die from stroke than white women. Compared to whites, blacks have a higher frequency of many known risk factors for stroke. These include high blood pressure, diabetes, smoking, excessive alcohol intake, heart disease, and sickle cell disease. The highest rate of all is found among African Americans living in the so-called Stroke Belt.

The **Stroke Belt** is an eleven-state area in the southeastern part of the United States, so named because of the high frequency of stroke occurring among all groups there. African Americans in particular who live in the Stroke Belt have some of the highest

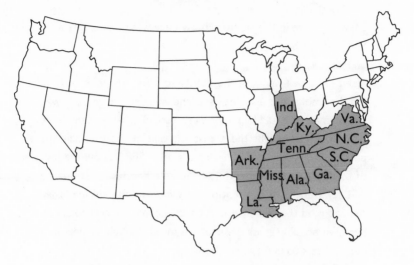

The stroke belt is an eleven-state area of the United States where the rate of stroke is high.

rates of high blood pressure and incidence of stroke seen anywhere in the country. Scientists think that environmental factors, including diet, probably play a role in this phenomenon. Obesity and the amount of the minerals (sodium, calcium, and potassium) that are commonly ingested in the food of that area may also play a role. Social factors, including feelings of stress and hostility (which are known to affect heart health), and a lack of access to quality health care may also contribute.

Lucy sat in the clinic waiting room, hoping that her mother's appointment wouldn't take much longer. She was already out of cigarettes. To pass the time, she glanced at the pamphlets that were lying on the low table next to her chair. Lucy started to flip through one published by the American Heart Association. The pamphlet was about stroke, which didn't interest her at all. Oh, well. She was about to put it down again when the phrase "stroke belt" caught her eye. It struck her funny. "Bible belt, I've heard of," she mused, "but stroke belt?"

It turned out that Louisiana, where she lived, was part of this so-called stroke belt. The term described a region of the southeastern United States where more strokes occurred than anywhere else in the country. Now Lucy was more interested. She read further.

Her curiosity soon grew into outright concern. She recognized in herself many of the risk factors for stroke. Not only did she smoke, but also, let's see, she was overweight, she was diabetic, and she had high blood pressure. The American Heart Association said right there that any one of those conditions put her at greater risk of having a stroke. She had quite a few of them. And she lived in the stroke belt, besides.

Lucy went to the receptionist's window and explained that she had read the AHA pamphlet and become concerned about her own possible stroke risk. She wanted to make an appointment to talk to her doctor about it.

A few days later, Lucy was back at the clinic, this time to see the doctor herself. "Am I going to have a stroke, doctor?" she asked worriedly.

"I'm afraid no one can predict with complete accuracy who will or will not have a stroke," her doctor told her. "However, there are things one can do to significantly reduce that risk, and that's what you should do, starting today. You do have a number of serious risk factors for stroke, Lucy. We can do something about some of them. I'm glad you came to see me," she added.

With her doctor's help, Lucy lowered her high blood pressure and got her diabetes under control for the first time in years. With the aid of a counselor, she also quit smoking and followed a slimming diet her doctor provided. Lucy learned healthful new ways to think about food and nutrition. Finally, she vowed to have regular checkups so that her doctor could keep up with any changes in her health before they became major problems.

A year later Lucy came across that AHA pamphlet she had read in the doctor's office. She sat down and reread it. She was pleased to note that she had eliminated or reduced many of her personal risk factors for stroke. She was no longer as afraid of stroke as she once was. Now she was doing the best she could to prevent it. Her doctor thought she was making good progress. Lucy realized she had a lot more energy these days, and she felt in control of her health for the first time in years.

Lucy felt quite confident about the beneficial changes she had introduced into her own life. In fact, she made a point of sharing what she had learned about stroke, risk factors, and prevention with her friends and fellow office workers. After all, they lived in the stroke belt, too.

She still thought "stroke belt" was a funny name.

Differences in the *types* of stroke that are most common to each ethnic group are also emerging. A better understanding of stroke incidence in this area is important. It eventually will help doctors diagnose strokes in progress more quickly and confidently. That ultimately means faster, better treatment for all people.

Doctors are finding that both African Americans and Asians tend to develop atherosclerotic deposits more frequently in the blood vessels inside the skull than elsewhere. These two groups also have a higher-than-average incidence of intracerebral hemorrhage and subarachnoid hemorrhage compared to whites. Compared to whites, both groups also tend to have lower-than-average incidences of atherosclerotic deposits in the carotid arteries of the neck. Both African Americans and Asians are highly susceptible to hypertension. But researchers aren't convinced that high blood pressure is the true cause for their findings, since the same pattern doesn't emerge among white hypertensives. Doctors think their findings may indicate that arteries in the brain narrow due to different causes and disease patterns than arteries elsewhere in the body. But more research will be needed to prove their hypothesis. In their continuing research, doctors are investigating the roles diet, cholesterol levels, and the prevalence and degree of high blood pressure may play in this condition.

Outcome *after* a stroke also may vary according to ethnic background and have implications for treatment. In a recent study, whites tended to show the highest stroke recurrence and death rates in the months just following a cerebral infarction. The next highest rate was among African Americans and then Hispanics. Six months after a stroke, however, the rate at which whites had another stroke or died stabilized. Black and Hispanic rates, though still lower than that of whites, continued to climb. If follow-up studies confirm these findings, it may mean that African Americans and Hispanics require medical attention longer than whites do after experiencing a stroke.

If research studies continue to confirm that racial differences do exist in stroke patterns, doctors will eventually have an even better understanding of the causes of different types of stroke. They will also have a better knowledge of how best to prevent them.

Diabetes Mellitus

Diabetes is the inability of the body to use glucose (sugar) properly. It most commonly appears in middle age and among overweight people. In its mild form, it can go undetected for years. Diabetes increases the risk of a number of other illnesses, including kidney disease, blindness, and nerve and blood vessel damage. Because the condition affects cholesterol and triglyceride levels in the blood, it also seriously increases the risk of cardiovascular disease, which in turn can cause thrombotic stroke. About 20 percent of people who have strokes have diabetes.

Diabetes is often found in persons who are obese, and have high blood pressure and other risk factors. Native Americans, Hispanics, and African Americans are more likely to develop diabetes than whites. The reason for this isn't entirely understood. One study has suggested that a high incidence of obesity among these ethnic groups may partially explain the statistics. (People are considered obese if they are more than 30 percent overweight.) Diabetes appears in midlife in many more women than men. This may be partially explained by the fact that women live longer. There are simply more women than men in an older population. Significantly, however, a large proportion of women are obese at the time of onset. The disease also seems to be more dangerous for women than for men.

To keep diabetes in check, a doctor may prescribe changes in eating habits, weight control, and exercise programs. If necessary, he may also prescribe drugs to control diabetes. Identifying the condition and controlling weight and blood pressure won't eliminate it. Unfortunately, it is a permanent condition. However, among diabetics, those whose diabetes is carefully controlled have a lower probability of having a stroke than do those whose diabetes is not controlled. And control of diabetes is important for another reason. Researchers now believe that unrecognized diabetes may result in a poor prognosis after stroke. If you have reason to suspect you might be diabetic or could develop the disease because of your risk factors or family background, be sure to discuss the matter with your doctor.

Pregnant women can also develop diabetes easily, and they should be monitored for any signs of the condition.

A Prior Stroke

Having had one stroke increases the likelihood of having another. One recent study that tracked ischemic stroke patients found that slightly more than one in six of them had second strokes within two years. Certain characteristics seemed to be associated with such an event, according to the report. These include elevated blood pressure, abnormal CT scans, or a history of diabetes mellitus.

The Treatable Risk Factors

If you do have risk factors you can't control, such as your age or the fact that you've already had a stroke, taking care of the risk factors you can control becomes even more important. Anyone who has risk factors that can be eliminated or reduced in some way ought to do so. The benefit is greater protection not only against possible stroke, but against a host of other potential health problems as well.

The following risk factors can be managed with a doctor's care.

Hypertension (High Blood Pressure)

Hypertension is the major risk factor associated with stroke.

Hypertension—abnormally high blood pressure—is an extremely damaging condition over time. It injures key organs, including the heart, and blood vessels in many parts of the body as well. Damage to these vital areas can lead to atherosclerosis and heart disease as well as stroke. If you have high blood pressure along with obesity, high blood cholesterol levels, or diabetes, or if you

MEDICATIONS FOR HIGH BLOOD PRESSURE

High blood pressure is one of the most important risk factors for stroke. Physicians will generally try to bring high blood pressure down into a normal range through diet and exercise first. Two avoidable risk factors contributing to hypertension are excessive salt intake and obesity. Controlling those factors can clear up a high blood pressure problem in many, if not most, people. But if nothing else works, or if your blood pressure must be brought down quickly, your doctor may prescribe medications.

The six types of antihypertensive medications described below can yield very different responses from person to person. If you're taking any of these prescribed medications, it is extremely important that you follow dosage instructions carefully—and that you stay on the medication as directed. Most people undergo trial periods with a few of them. Then they stay with the one that is most effective and has the fewest side effects.

Diuretics. These rid the body of excess salts (especially sodium chloride) and water. High sodium in the diet can contribute to high blood pressure.

Beta blockers. These drugs affect blood pressure by a number of mechanisms.

Sympathetic nerve inhibitors. The so-called sympathetic nerves control many automatic responses in the body, including those having to do with constricting the arteries. (Narrower blood vessels raise blood pressure.) Sympathetic nerve inhibitors are a class of drugs that block messages from the brain to constrict vessels.

Vasodilators. This group of drugs works by relaxing muscles in the artery walls, causing them to widen, or dilate.

Angiotensin converting enzyme (ACE) inhibitors. The angiotensin converting enzyme, when released, results in constricted arteries. ACE inhibitors interfere with that job to keep arteries dilated and blood pressure down.

Calcium antagonists (calcium channel blockers). These drugs work by reducing the person's heart rate and relaxing the blood vessels.

also smoke, your risk of heart attack or stroke increases several times.

More than 62 million Americans over the age of six are hypertensive. Almost half of them don't even realize it and therefore aren't controlling their condition. That's at least 29 million people who today are needlessly at risk for stroke and other disease. Hypertension usually causes no symptoms. So people can be hypertensive for years without knowing it—until serious damage is already done, including atherosclerosis and stroke. That fact has earned hypertension the nickname of "the silent killer." On the brighter side, however, high blood pressure is easy to identify in a quick, painless test. Every year more people are recognizing the importance of keeping their high blood pressure under control. Stroke incidence and mortality are declining as a result. But there is still a long way to go before everyone who is at risk is identified. The evidence is clear: Taking care of high blood pressure is good for your health.

Joe could hardly remember a time when he wasn't working hard as a house framer. It was exhausting labor, but, at fifty, he felt as fit as he had at thirty. He was particularly proud of the fact that he often beat his younger friends at racquetball. Joe had been athletic and a competitor his whole life.

So, when a routine checkup showed he had developed hypertension, or high blood pressure, he was a little disappointed. He had expected all of his medical tests to come back perfect. Dr. Freeman prescribed medication for the condition. He also told Joe to cut out the salty foods and to check back in six months. Joe thought that was going a little too far. How important could this hypertension be? he thought to himself. I don't smoke or drink or anything. I haven't been sick in years. I feel absolutely great. Never better, in fact.

Still, for a short while he tried to follow his doctor's directions. He bought the prescribed medication, and he even took it—for a few weeks. Then he forgot a couple of times. It seemed like he just kept forgetting. He was not used to taking medication. After all, he felt the same whether he took it or not. It couldn't be doing any good, he decided. The same went for salted food. He tried to cut back, but everything he liked seemed to have salt in it, anyway. So why bother?

Joe reverted to his old habits fairly quickly. At first he felt a little guilty about that. But he soon forgot about his high blood pressure entirely. Six months after his first visit, he canceled the follow-up appointment. A conflict had come up. Joe forgot to reschedule.

When the flu brought Joe back to his doctor's office a year later, Dr. Freeman took Joe's blood pressure again. It was still quite high because Joe hadn't followed through on any of the remedies originally prescribed. After the exam, the doctor ushered Joe into his office.

"What's the problem?" Dr. Freeman asked. "Have you had trouble keeping your blood pressure down since you were diagnosed? According to my notes, you canceled your follow-up and never rescheduled. Joe, this is extremely important. Have you kept up with the medications and cut your salt intake?"

Joe felt a little silly in the face of his doctor's obvious concern. He admitted that he hadn't taken care of his high blood pressure because he didn't really see what the fuss was about. "I feel fine, doctor," he protested.

"Listen, Joe, you aren't fine," Dr. Freeman said emphatically. "I guess I didn't make myself clear the first time around. Did you know your condition is sometimes called 'the silent killer'? What's most dangerous about it is the fact that many of its victims show no symptoms—none—until they have a major stroke. That could be you, Joe, unless you follow my instructions to the letter. You must bring your blood pressure back into a normal range and keep it there!

"Ignoring the problem doesn't make it go away. Unfortunately, it simply sets the stage for a serious medical crisis later on. I can't emphasize it enough, Joe," Dr. Freeman continued. "You're a male, you're getting older, and you have very high blood pressure. You have three risk factors for stroke right there. You can control only one of those things: your high blood pressure. So it is extremely important that you do so. Any questions?"

Joe had to admit his doctor was persuasive. He understood his condition much better now, he told Dr. Freeman. "Let's start again," Joe said. And they did.

Some factors that contribute to the development of hypertension can't be changed. These include heredity, race, and age. But others can be controlled successfully, especially with a doctor's help. People with high blood pressure should maintain a low-fat, low-salt diet, keep their weight within a normal range, exercise regularly, and drink alcohol in moderation, if at all. Often these steps alone take care of the problem. Sometimes, however, lifestyle changes by themselves aren't enough. In these cases, medication under a doctor's supervision usually brings high blood pressure under control.

Effective treatment for hypertension is available, but it requires your active participation to work. Have your blood pressure checked regularly, and take responsibility for bringing it down to a normal range if necessary.

When is blood pressure considered "too high"? How can you tell if you are hypertensive? Because high blood pressure has no symptoms, doctors rely on a simple blood pressure test to detect it.

Blood Pressure Defined

Blood pressure is a measurement of the force of blood as it is pumped through the body's circulatory system. A blood pressure reading actually takes two measurements. Both are expressed as millimeters of mercury (mm Hg). One is the **systolic pressure,** which is the maximum pressure created as the heart beats. The second is **diastolic pressure,** which reflects the minimum pressure of blood flow, taken when the heart is at rest between beats. Systolic pressure is noted as the top number on a blood pressure reading. Diastolic pressure is represented by the bottom number. **A blood pressure measurement with a systolic above 140 mm Hg or a diastolic over 90 mm Hg, taken on several consecutive readings, is considered high and should be controlled.**

Even if you have no other risk factors, a high blood pressure is a very significant risk factor. A measurement of 160/95 mm Hg puts you at more than *three* times the risk of stroke compared to a person whose blood pressure is 120/90 mm Hg, a reading within the normal-to-low range. Don't be complacent if you are told you have "borderline" hypertension, which falls below 160 mm Hg and above 120 mm Hg systolic readings. Almost three-quarters of all hypertensives fall into this category, and they too have a substantially higher stroke risk compared to those with lower readings.

How Is Blood Pressure Measured?

Blood pressure is measured by a quick, painless test using a medical instrument called a sphygmomanometer. A rubber cuff is wrapped around a person's upper arm and inflated. When the cuff is inflated, it compresses a large artery in the arm. This momentarily stops the flow of blood.

Next, air in the cuff is released, and the person measuring the blood pressure listens with a stethoscope. When the blood starts to pulse through the artery, it makes a sound. Sounds continue to be heard until pressure in the artery exceeds the pressure in the cuff.

While the person listens and watches the sphygmomanometer gauge, he records two measurements. The **systolic** pressure is the pressure of blood flow when the heart beats (the pressure when the first sound is heard). The **diastolic** pressure is the pressure between heartbeats (the pressure when the last sound is heard). Blood pressure is measured in millimeters of mercury, which is abbreviated "mm Hg."

A typical blood pressure reading for an adult might be 130/80 mm Hg, although readings vary depending on age and other factors. (Normal blood pressure is defined by a range of values, so don't be alarmed if your own reading is somewhat higher or lower than the example given above.) The first, larger number is the systolic pressure. The second is the diastolic pressure.

The harder it is for blood to flow, the higher the numbers will be.

Simply put, the higher your blood pressure, the greater your risk of stroke.

What Causes High Blood Pressure and Who Is Susceptible?

Unfortunately, doctors don't know the exact causes of high blood pressure. They know only the factors that influence the condition. There is no "cure" for hypertension. Only careful control of high blood pressure is effective.

Some groups are more prone to developing hypertension than others. Age, race, and heredity all play a part. Pregnant women are at greater risk of becoming hypertensive than other women.

In this country, African Americans, Asians, Puerto Ricans, Cuban Americans, and Hispanics are more often hypertensive than other groups. Deaths related to high blood pressure are at least three to five times more frequent in African Americans than in whites, for example. The role race plays in the appearance of high blood pressure isn't fully understood.

A strong inverse relationship, however, has been detected between the prevalence of high blood pressure and socioeconomic class. The lower one's socioeconomic standing, the higher the incidence of high blood pressure. That strongly suggests that environment is an important factor in the appearance of high blood pressure among minority groups in this country. People at the lower end of the socioeconomic scale tend to have a great deal of stress and instability in their lives. They also tend to have less education and face more unemployment than others. These conditions could in turn promote behaviors that are known risk factors for hypertension. These risk factors include a poor diet, smoking, excessive drinking, and inadequate exercise. More study will be necessary, however, to confirm or refute this hypothesis.

The Special Case of African Americans and Hypertension. High blood pressure is a major health problem for African Americans. It is the number-one preventable cause of death for this group. More than 30 percent of black adults have hypertension. For African Americans over sixty-five years old, the rate approaches 80 percent. High blood pressure also develops at an earlier age in blacks than in whites, and when it appears, it tends to be more severe. African Americans have almost twice the number of strokes as whites do from causes traced to high blood pressure.

Yet as sensitive as this population appears to be to high blood pressure, there may be more to the story. The susceptibility to developing the disease may remain dormant until triggered by various factors. These include weight gain, excessive salt intake, alcohol consumption, or lack of exercise. There is evidence that prevention of these health problems can make an important difference in whether or not an African American develops high blood pressure. But prevention must begin as early in life as possible. Medical intervention alone is seldom as effective as prevention.

Older People and High Blood Pressure. Older people are also likely to have unchecked hypertension, or high blood pressure.

Most people over sixty-five years old have this condition, whose incidence increases with age. More older blacks, especially black women, are likely to be hypertensive than older whites. High blood pressure is so common among older people that doctors used to consider it a natural consequence of aging, and so they didn't treat it aggressively. Now, because therapy is low risk and quite beneficial, older people are routinely treated for high blood pressure when necessary, as they should be. The risk of stroke or other cardiovascular illness is very high for this group if high blood pressure is left untreated.

Women and High Blood Pressure. High blood pressure has often been attributed to the stresses of modern living. Many people think of hypertension as a "man's disease." That's just not true. Women, too, develop the disease in significant numbers. Often they go untreated simply because they never get checked for it. In fact, more than a fourth of all women in this country between the ages of eighteen and seventy-four have high blood pressure. An even greater percentage of black women are at risk of having high blood pressure.

Women who have never been hypertensive before can develop the condition during pregnancy, especially in the last three months before giving birth. Left untreated, it endangers both mother and baby. Hypertensive women who take oral contraceptives (the "Pill") are at a much higher risk for stroke than those who don't. If you are taking oral contraceptives, discuss this with your doctor and be sure to have your blood pressure checked regularly. You may wish to consider another form of birth control. Those hypertensive women who smoke in addition to taking oral contraceptives are upping their odds for stroke even more dramatically. The message is clear. If you smoke, STOP!

High blood pressure is most likely to appear in women after menopause. More than half of all women between the ages of fifty-five and sixty-four have high blood pressure. After sixty-five, more than two-thirds are affected. In fact, after age sixty-five, women become more likely than men to develop the disease.

Hypertension and Lifestyle

Behavioral factors also play a significant part in the development of high blood pressure. Anyone who is more than 30 percent over-weight, consumes a high-salt diet, drinks excessive amounts of alcohol, and doesn't get adequate exercise is setting up the right conditions for high blood pressure. All of these things have been clearly associated with hypertension and in turn with stroke. Make no mistake, all of these things can be controlled. But it's up to *you* to make it happen! Today more than three-fifths of all hypertensives in this country aren't on any therapy at all for their condition. More than a fifth are on inadequate therapy. Just 11 percent are getting the right therapy to keep their hypertension in check.

If you don't know whether you are hypertensive or not, check it out. If you know you are, talk with your doctor and set up a program for controlling it. This program should be tailored to your individual needs. Simply adjusting your diet and getting enough exercise may be all that is necessary to get the results you want. If high blood pressure stubbornly persists, your doctor may decide to try medical therapy as well. Do whatever it takes. When hypertension is treated, stroke risk goes down.

Even if you aren't hypertensive, it makes sense to follow a program that keeps your risk of ever developing the condition as low as possible. The evidence is clear. Following a low-salt diet, maintaining an ideal weight, cutting out excessive alcohol consumption, and getting enough exercise make sound sense for everyone.

How Can Salt Intake Affect My Condition?

Sodium is a mineral essential to health. It contributes to the balance of the water in the **vascular** system in the body. Most sodium in the diet comes from the compound sodium chloride, or common table salt. The average American consumes one or two teaspoons of salt daily, or 6 to 18 grams. But the body only needs a fraction of that—about half a gram—every day. Besides table salt, some other common sources of sodium include: monosodium glutamate (MSG), baking soda, baking powder, and over-the-counter drugs.

Unfortunately, the mechanism linking high sodium intake to high blood pressure isn't fully understood yet. But the link, whatever it is, is real. Sodium intake affects blood pressure levels in about three-fifths of all hypertensives.

A possible explanation for this situation is that eating salty foods triggers thirst and the drinking of fluids. This leads to an increase in the blood volume of the body. That increase means the heart has to pump harder to meet the new output, and blood pressure rises. The new, higher pressure in turn affects the kidneys, which have to filter more salt and water as a result. Now, because input must equal output in this closed system, a higher level of salt and water is present in the body. This brings us back to the heart, which starts the pumping process all over again at a higher pressure than before.

Practically all foods contain some sodium naturally. Simply by decreasing or eliminating salt added to food and by staying away from salty prepared foods, many people find that their blood pressure comes down to normal levels. Some people are more sensitive to salt than others, however. These people in addition may need to watch their weight, cut out drinking alcoholic beverages, and take prescribed medication under a doctor's supervision to get the same benefit.

Heart Disease

Heart disease is an undeniable risk factor for stroke, especially ischemic stroke. Those who have some form of heart disease are twice as likely to have a stroke as those without it. In fact, up to a fifth of all ischemic strokes occur in people who have already developed some form of heart disease. The reasons for this vary depending on the type of heart disease involved. Myocardial infarctions, or heart attacks, damage the heart and create emboli. These emboli subsequently travel through the arteries into the brain. There they get stuck and block further blood flow, causing a cerebral infarction. Artificial heart valves also carry a significant risk of sending emboli to the brain in the postoperative period, especially in the first two and a half years. (By the third year after surgery, however, the risk begins to diminish.) There are other significant heart ailments relating to stroke. These include congestive heart failure, rheumatic heart disease, atrial fibrillation, and other cardiac arrhythmias.

Stopping or never starting cigarette smoking and controlling high blood cholesterol levels and high blood pressure all reduce the risk of heart disease and therefore the risk of stroke. Cigarette smoking is also a direct risk factor for stroke as well.

Transient Ischemic Attack, or TIA

A TIA is an urgent medical matter in its own right and should be treated accordingly. It is also a major risk factor for an ischemic stroke. Possibly up to a fifth of all ischemic strokes are preceded by

TIAs, but the hard numbers aren't known. Doctors do know that up to one-third of people who have had a TIA will have a stroke within the following four or five years.

The risk of stroke is greatest in the first month following a TIA: One-fifth of all subsequent strokes occur then. Half will have occurred within the first year. After that, stroke incidence drops off. Some people experience more than one TIA over time, without having a full-blown stroke at all. That doesn't mean their risk of having a stroke eventually is any less than it is for others, however. Their most recent TIA episode is still considered a major risk factor. No episode of TIA should ever be ignored. Anyone who experiences one should be evaluated by his doctor as soon as possible. The doctor will try to find the cause of the TIA and may prescribe one or more medications.

Lifestyle Choices

Medical advancements have impressively improved our odds of avoiding stroke by controlling some of the major risk factors for the disease. But it's becoming ever clearer that the choices we make in our lifestyles have an equally significant role to play in that effort. Smoking is a primary risk factor for stroke. There are other "lifestyle" risk factors that are considered **secondary risk factors.** They themselves do not cause stroke, but they influence the development of diseases that do. Often they are guilty by association to more than one health problem. Getting rid of them very often not only improves your chances against having a stroke, but helps prevent other problems as well, including heart disease and adult-onset diabetes. By stopping smoking, for example, you greatly improve the odds that you will never have a stroke. You also have a much better chance of avoiding heart attack, lung cancer, high blood pressure, and a variety of other associated illnesses. Not a bad tradeoff!

Cigarette Smoking

Cigarette smoking has been called the most important preventable cause of premature death in the United States. Long associated with cancer, smoking has equally strong links to a variety of other diseases. These include stroke, atherosclerosis, and heart disease. (As we have seen, both atherosclerosis and heart disease are important risk factors for stroke.) An estimated 450,000 deaths are attributed to smoking every year. Surprisingly to some, most of these deaths result from cardiovascular diseases, not cancer. By quitting smoking, however, former puffers can turn their odds around dramatically. Make no mistake: The consequences of smoking are real—and so are the benefits of quitting.

How Does Smoking Affect My Chances of Having a Stroke?

About *four thousand* substances have been identified in cigarette smoke. This smoke winds up in the lungs of those exposed to it and then his bloodstream. Of these, nicotine and carbon monoxide seem to do the most damage. **Nicotine** affects the heart and blood vessels by causing vessels to constrict. This increases one's blood pressure and heart rate. When **carbon monoxide** enters the bloodstream, it "bumps" oxygen needed by the heart and all the other parts of the body. Because less oxygen is available to the body, the heart has to work harder to make up the difference.

Smoking low-tar and low-nicotine cigarettes does *not* decrease one's risk of heart disease, however. The reason? Smokers often wind up smoking more of these "lighter" cigarettes and inhaling them more deeply. They actually get more smoke in their lungs and more of the noxious compounds they are trying to avoid. The people around them are exposed to more smoke as well.

Thousands of other unwelcome substances enter the bloodstream when people are exposed to smoke. These, too, are damaging, probably injuring vessel walls as they scrape by. Tobacco smoke also causes existing blood platelets to become stickier than normal and to cluster. The thicker blood that results can injure the vessels it flows through. Both of these damaging conditions allow more blood cholesterol to affix to roughened vessel walls as plaques, introducing the right conditions for atherosclerosis. How much one is exposed to smoke and for how long has been found to influence directly the thickness of plaque that clogs arteries supplying the brain. **People exposed to tobacco smoke—their own or someone else's—develop atherosclerosis more frequently and more severely than people not exposed to it.**

Tobacco smoke has a terrible effect on the body's vascular system. It compounds the bad effects of other diseases on the body as well.

Numbers Don't Lie: Smoking and Stroke. Smoking—whether active or passive—is clearly an important risk factor for stroke, as well as other diseases. But how great a risk is it? The facts are undeniable: The risk is *very* high.

Men who smoke have fully a 40 percent greater chance of having a debilitating stroke than those who do not smoke. Women smokers are even worse off: They have a 60 percent greater chance of having a stroke compared to nonsmoking women.

A recent study found that overall, smokers seem to run more than four times the risk of a subarachnoid hemorrhage (SAH) than nonsmokers. And this risk seems to rise with how much they smoke. SAH is a relatively rare type of stroke that is also very difficult to treat. It is most commonly associated with younger people, and with women more than men. Women smokers appear to be more sensitive to smoking's adverse effects than men. When women were separated from the whole population of the study group, their baseline risk rose to slightly more than four and a half times that of nonsmokers. Women who smoke are also much less likely to quit than men who do.

This same study found that heavy smokers were worse off than average smokers, carrying eleven times the stroke risk of nonsmokers. (Heavy cigarette smoking is considered a pack a day or more.) And while a regular exercise program seemed to decrease the risk of SAH by 40 percent for nonsmokers in the group, smokers benefitted much less from the practice.

Smoking has an especially toxic effect on women who also take oral contraceptives. These women are an astronomical twenty-two times more likely to have a stroke than their nonsmoking peers who use other forms of birth control.

Okie was a typical young mother. She juggled the demands of a marriage, two kids, and a job. She had very little time to herself, and she had learned to economize wherever she could.

Medical checkups, unfortunately, were one of the places

where Okie economized on time and money. As long as she was "up and running," as she put it, Okie steered clear of her doctor. She hadn't been sick in years, or to a doctor in all that time. She figured that, at thirty-five, she was too young to bother if she didn't absolutely have to.

Okie had started smoking five years before when she went to work at the family store. She knew smoking two to three packs a day wasn't good for her, but she really enjoyed smoking. She hadn't smoked during her pregnancies. Besides, she had always been a healthy person. She figured she'd have to quit smoking someday—maybe when she turned fifty.

Unknowingly, however, Okie had activated a medical time bomb several years before. It was one a doctor could have spotted and addressed immediately. She had been taking oral contraceptives for ten years, since the birth of her second child. She had renewed her prescription automatically at a pharmacy every six months. Okie knew millions of women were on the Pill, as she was. She never worried about it. Most of those millions of women didn't also smoke heavily, as Okie did. She didn't realize that the two practices were particularly dangerous to her health when combined.

Okie had started smoking after going on the Pill. Consequently, she hadn't been warned about a stroke risk when she originally settled on this birth control method with her doctor. Having a stroke was about the furthest thing from Okie's mind. She'd never heard of a person her age having one. Besides, she had enough to think about, between chasing after her kids and working at the store.

Both the Pill she took and the cigarettes she smoked had side effects that aggravated Okie's risk of stroke. Cigarettes, of course, were a health risk for a number of reasons, not all of which had to do with either stroke or the Pill. When smoking and the Pill were combined, however, the dynamics of the stroke-risk equation changed dramatically. Despite her age and otherwise healthy constitution, Okie now had twenty-two times the risk of stroke as another woman her age who did not smoke or take the Pill.

Okie badly needs to see her doctor to defuse this time bomb, but she doesn't know it. She should quit smoking. If she chooses not to give up smoking, she must get a new form of birth control to improve her stroke risk profile. Sadly, until she does she is on a collision course with stroke.

Where's the Good News? Unfortunately, if you smoke, there is no good news—unless you stop the habit. There *is* a reward for quitting, and it's an impressive one. Those who stop smoking permanently enjoy a dramatically improved health profile. Within a year of quitting, a former smoker's risk of stroke begins to fall. Ten years later, his risk is basically the same as that of a similar nonsmoker.

More and more people in this country are choosing to give up or never start smoking. This is true for women as well as men. Habits are changing. The message that smoking is bad medicine is getting across. Still, an estimated 55 million people continue to smoke despite the powerful evidence against it. And that's 55 million too many.

The evidence is clear: If you smoke, STOP. Your doctor can help. And if you don't smoke, don't start.

Atherosclerosis

Arteriosclerosis is commonly called "hardening of the arteries." One form is atherosclerosis, a slow, progressive disease that causes fatty deposits and other materials to build up in the arteries. The term itself comes from the Greek words *athero,* which means "gruel" or "paste," and *sclerosis,* which means "hardness." Atherosclerosis affects large- and medium-sized arteries. It is one of the most common adult health disorders and a major cause of cardiovascular disease. Only a tiny fraction of those who live into their seventies are without significant atherosclerotic vascular disease. Let's take a closer look at this disease.

Atherosclerosis usually starts in the aorta. It advances into the coronary arteries next and eventually reaches the cerebral arteries. This progression may partially explain why more strokes occur among older people than any other age group. Men and women progress differently with this disease: Atherosclerosis in the cerebral arteries generally develops about ten years later in women than it does in men. Where the deposits accumulate also varies among individuals.

Scientists do not know the causes of atherosclerosis. They do know that some factors contribute to its development, however. These are high blood pressure, elevated cholesterol levels, and diabetes. All of these affect the vascular system and may accelerate and accentuate the development of the disease. Cigarette smoking also contributes to the formation of atherosclerotic deposits.

Abnormal levels of fats (cholesterol or triglycerides) or other substances carried in the bloodstream may irritate or damage the vessel walls. (Triglycerides are the chemical form in which most fats exist.) Irregularities in the vessel walls themselves may likewise allow fats and other substances in the blood to catch instead of being swept along. However it initially happens, when the blood vessel is damaged, atherosclerosis can get started.

When the artery is damaged, the arterial cells can separate from the inner wall of the blood vessel. This allows other materials to attach to the connective tissue (collagen) and smooth muscle tissue underneath. Blood platelets collect on the collagen around the wound first. Then fats, cholesterol, cellular waste products, calcium, and fibrin (a clotting substance)—all carried in the blood—catch along the rough, damaged inner wall of the artery over time. These substances accumulate on the smooth muscle cells, irritating them, and the cell wall thickens in response.

Scarring occurs after this, due to the irritation of and injury caused by the deposits left along the artery. From this scarring, a plaque develops. Over time, the artery may narrow as the plaque builds up. Less blood can pass because the diameter of the artery decreases. Plaque may partially or completely block the blood flow through an artery. Or it may cause the vessel to which it has attached to hemorrhage, creating blood clots.

Atherosclerosis can cause a stroke in two ways. If some part of the rough plaque is detached and washed into the bloodstream, or a blood clot breaks away from it, an embolus is born. That embolus may travel to the brain, causing an infarction. Or a blood clot may develop as a result of the plaque. If the clot closes off the vessel to blood flow entirely, a thrombotic stroke occurs.

Elevated Blood Cholesterol and Lipids (Fats)

The exact role of elevated blood lipids (or blood fats) as a risk factor for stroke remains unclear, but a link is there. It increases the risk of heart disease and stroke because it accelerates the development of atherosclerosis. Cholesterol, a fatlike substance the body manufactures, is also found in animal products like meat, eggs, and dairy products. Saturated fats, however, which are found in a number of other sources, tend to raise the body's blood cholesterol level, too. Examples of these are animal fats and tropical oils (such as palm and coconut).

CHOLESTEROL LEVEL	CLASSIFICATION
Less than 200 mg/dl	Desirable
200–239 mg/dl	Borderline High
240 mg/dl or greater	Undesirable

Scientists have established guidelines for blood cholesterol levels that relate to this risk. Cholesterol is measured in milligrams per deciliter of blood (mg/dl).

DESIRABLE BLOOD LIPOPROTEIN LEVELS

High-density lipoprotein (HDL) should be above 35 mg/dl
Low-density lipoprotein (LDL) should be below 130 mg/dl

Note: The cholesterol levels above were derived from studies of men only. The most beneficial levels for women may be slightly different, but no tests are available yet to indicate what they might be.

The higher your blood cholesterol level, the greater your chance of developing atherosclerosis. In addition to heart attack, atherosclerosis can cause stroke when it develops in the brain or in the arteries leading to the brain. Have your cholesterol level tested every five years if it is less than 200 mg/dl. If your total cholesterol is higher than that, be sure to discuss your cholesterol level with your doctor. You should also get breakdowns that reflect the levels of the two major components of cholesterol. These are **high-density lipoprotein (HDL)** and **low-density lipoprotein (LDL).**

Lipoproteins carry cholesterol in the bloodstream. There is evidence that HDL, sometimes called the "good" cholesterol, is associated with a decreased risk of heart disease. It may be protective because it carries cholesterol out of the arteries to the liver, where it is eliminated. Scientists think LDL, on the other hand, tends to retain cholesterol in the body. If there is an imbalance of cholesterol in the bloodstream, LDL may be responsible for allowing the excess to collect on artery walls.

For most people, following a low-fat diet, participating in regular physical activity, and not smoking can adequately lower their LDL and raise their HDL levels. Some, however, have an inherited tendency toward high blood cholesterol levels. For these people, diet changes alone may not do the trick. Their doctors may prescribe drug therapy along with diet changes.

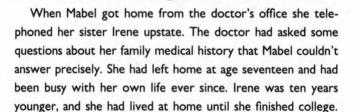

When Mabel got home from the doctor's office she telephoned her sister Irene upstate. The doctor had asked some questions about her family medical history that Mabel couldn't answer precisely. She had left home at age seventeen and had been busy with her own life ever since. Irene was ten years younger, and she had lived at home until she finished college. Maybe she would know some answers.

"Hi, Irene, it's me," she began. "Look, I saw my doctor today. . . . No, I'm OK, it's just that we got to talking. . . . He thinks I need to lose fifty pounds. That's not the first time I've heard that, but that's not why I'm calling."

"You sound worried," Irene said.

"He asked me some questions about our family medical history. Irene, I just can't remember details from that far back. Do you know whether Mother or Dad had high blood pressure? . . . Oh, they did?" Mabel sighed. She had just learned she had high blood pressure, too.

Irene remembered both of their parents having high blood

pressure. In fact, their father had taken medication for the condition, she told Mabel.

"What about diabetes? Do you remember anybody in our family being diabetic?" Mabel asked.

Irene thought. "Not Mother or Dad," she said slowly. "Come to think of it, Grandma developed diabetes when she was older—about what, sixty or so? Something like that."

Mabel didn't answer. She would be sixty next month.

"Mabel, are you there?"

"Yes, I'm here," Mabel answered quietly.

"Why all the questions, anyway? Are you sure you're telling me everything? C'mon, Sis, talk to me," Irene encouraged.

Mabel told Irene that her doctor was concerned about her weight and high blood pressure. He thought that she had a good chance of developing diabetes, too, especially if it was in the family background. And he had wanted to know whether high blood pressure ran in the family. If it did, that meant Mabel's condition might not completely respond to changes in diet alone. He might need to think about prescribing medication in order to keep it under control.

"Do you have high blood pressure, Irene?" Mabel asked. "Apparently if either or both parents have it, their children may be more likely to develop it, too."

"So far, my blood pressure has always been normal," Irene assured her sister.

"That's good. Anyway, between being overweight, hypertensive, and apparently a candidate for diabetes, I have something else to worry about. My doctor says I have a much higher than normal stroke risk right now, too," Mabel said.

"A stroke! That's serious. What can you do?" Irene asked.

"Well, first, I need to get my blood pressure down. I have to cut out the sodium in my diet. If that doesn't work, I will need to take medication. My doctor wants to keep a close watch on me. He says I need to be monitored for diabetes. He says if I can lose this weight and watch my diet, maybe I won't develop diabetes."

"I'm so sorry to hear all this, Mabel. Is there anything I can do?"

"Just be your usual encouraging self. I know it's going to be hard for me to make these changes, but I am going to give it my best shot."

"Sounds like you have excellent incentive for that, Mabel," her sister observed. "Will it keep you motivated?"

"I think so. It still won't be easy to lose weight. You should see the diet my doctor gave me. It makes perfect sense! You know, I have tried about a hundred fad diets and every one of them failed. This diet is different. It just recommends eating moderate amounts of foods that are good for me. I think I can do it. It helps to remember why it's important," Mabel commented.

"That sounds great. I know you can do it. Look, I'll call you again next week to see how you're doing. Say, I have an idea. Let's get together in the city next month—for your birthday. Can you get away for a long weekend?"

"I don't know, Irene." She really didn't feel in a very festive mood.

"At least say you'll try!" Irene pleaded.

"OK, OK." Irene had always been persuasive.

"Good. After all, we haven't celebrated a birthday together in a long time. I think it's high time we did! I'll see what I can arrange."

"Thanks, Sis," Mabel said.

"Bye! See you soon!" Irene said cheerfully.

Alcohol Consumption

Heavy drinking, including binge drinking, appears to be strongly associated with stroke. More than two alcoholic drinks a day raises blood pressure levels, and high blood pressure is a powerful risk factor for stroke. There is also some evidence that people who completely abstain from drinking alcohol have a lower risk of heart disease—another stroke risk factor—than do moderate drinkers.

The American Heart Association recommends drinking no more than the equivalent of one ounce of pure alcohol per day, if you wish to drink at all. That equals 2 ounces of 100-proof spirits, OR 3 ounces of 80-proof spirits OR 8 ounces of wine OR 24 ounces of beer.

Obesity

Obesity is a significant secondary risk factor for stroke. Obesity is defined as being more than 30 percent overweight. Obese people are much more likely than their thinner friends to become hypertensive or diabetic and to develop heart disease. These are three primary risk factors for stroke. But even without those other risk factors present, they are more likely to develop stroke than those who aren't so overweight. Sometimes people inherit a tendency toward obesity. Women are especially susceptible to developing these dangerous conditions if they are seriously overweight. This is especially true of African American women.

Differences in types of obesity are determined by how people become overweight—where they put on that weight and how rapidly they gain it. Because of these differences, the true risk ratio of obesity to stroke isn't precisely known. It may vary according to the prominence of these factors in each individual. We do know that people within a normal weight range have an easier time controlling existing high blood pressure and diabetes. And people with a genetic predisposition to high blood pressure and diabetes may be able to delay their onset indefinitely by maintaining a proper weight.

Besides reducing one's stroke risk, losing excess weight and maintaining a low-fat diet can bring a number of other health benefits. The best way to lose weight successfully over the long term is simply to eat less and exercise more. If your eating habits aren't what they should be, your doctor can provide you with a sensible long-term diet plan and get you started.

Exercise

Regular exercise bestows health benefits no matter what your age. It helps fight heart disease and other conditions related to stroke. These include high blood pressure, obesity, and undesirable blood cholesterol levels. (Exercise increases the body's output of HDL— the "good" cholesterol.) By helping to prevent heart attack, exercise may reduce the risk of some kinds of embolic stroke.

Exercising moderately three times a week for fifteen to thirty minutes is enough to give your system the workout it needs and provide you with more energy. Be sure to check with your doctor before starting a new exercise program.

Oral Contraceptives

There is some conflicting evidence right now as to whether or not oral contraceptives increase a woman's likelihood of stroke. Some studies have shown that using birth control pills tends to raise one's blood pressure, as well as blood cholesterol and blood sugar levels. The Pill may also contribute to the formation of blood clots, especially in those women who already have some heart or vessel disease. The catch is, most of these findings are based on earlier studies made with a high-estrogen version of the Pill that is no longer used. The new types so far seem not to increase heart attack risk *unless* a woman also smokes or has other contributing risk factors. More studies will be needed to prove whether a link exists between today's lower-estrogen oral contraceptives and stroke.

If you are considering this form of birth control, you should first discuss with your doctor the risks and the benefits of the Pill compared to other methods. A discussion should include an evaluation of your medical history, need for birth control, age, and whether or not you smoke. Your doctor should check your blood pressure before putting you on the Pill, and you should get it checked every six months thereafter to be sure it remains within a normal range.

Right now, women in their twenties are considered at low risk of developing stroke from the Pill (if no other risk factors are present). This risk rises somewhat for women in their thirties, and probably these women should think about trying other methods. At forty years old and above, however, women should probably avoid the Pill altogether in favor of another birth control strategy.

There is no controversy, however, on one matter: **If you smoke and take the Pill, you are definitely increasing your risk of stroke.** If you smoke, stop before going on the Pill or choose another form of birth control.

Estrogen Replacement Therapy (ERT)

Doctors believe that estrogen protects against heart disease. As with the Pill, earlier studies indicated that women who were on ERT had a much greater risk of stroke than those who weren't. But today estrogen replacement therapy gives women less estrogen and adds progestin, a synthetic female hormone, to the mix. Recent studies indicate that this version of ERT actually *reduces* stroke by half in postmenopausal women. Why the difference? One reason is that the earlier studies involved higher estrogen dosages and no progestin at all. Another is that the earlier studies monitored women who were older, smoked, and already had some form of heart disease. Still, more studies specifically targeted to stroke risk are called for before doctors will be sure of the exact relationship between ERT and stroke.

Special Risk Groups

Sickle Cell Anemia

Sickle cell anemia is a genetic disease affecting the red blood cells. Normally round, cells affected by this disease collapse into a sickle shape because of an abnormal form of hemoglobin they contain. The condition is most common in African Americans and Hispanics. It is highly associated with stroke risk, especially in children. About one in fourteen of those with the disease will develop a stroke at some point in life. (Sickle cell trait without any anemia is not as strong a predictor of stroke.)

Lainie's seven-year-old son, Alex, had been playing outside after dinner when his best friend, Dwight, came rushing into the house. Come quick, he said. Alex had "stopped running" and "fallen down." He wasn't moving, the boy added fearfully.

Lainie rushed into the yard and scooped up her son in her arms. "I have to take Alex to the hospital right now, Dwight," she said. "It's OK. You were right to find me. I need you to run home now. Tell your mom what happened, and tell her to call Alex's dad at work, OK?" She was already on her way to the car.

At the emergency room, Alex was given a number of tests, and his mother was asked a lot of questions about his medical background. During this time Marvin joined his wife at the hospital. The African-American couple wondered, could this sudden illness have anything to do with their son's sickle cell disease?

A short while later, when the test results came in, Lainie

and Marvin learned that the answer to that question was yes. Their son Alex had had a thrombotic stroke—which was strongly associated with sickle cell disease, especially in children. The attending doctor gravely told them that Alex's condition had stabilized, but he was still unconscious. For the time being, they would all have to wait and see.

———————————————

Sickle cell anemia is the most common cause of stroke in children, and thromboembolic stroke is the most common type of stroke for this group. Adults with sickle cell anemia, however, tend to have hemorrhagic stroke. There is a high probability of recurrent stroke for those with sickle cell anemia, especially within the first thirty-six months after the initial stroke.

Scientists used to attribute the high stroke probability for this group to the presence of the abnormally shaped red blood cells, which they believed could clump together and clog blood vessels. But recently at least one researcher has suspected the problem may lie with abnormally narrowed arteries that many sickle cell stroke patients seem to have inside the brain. If these findings are borne out, in the future it may be advisable to screen sickle cell patients for this problem using transcranial Doppler (TCD). Blood flowing through narrowed arteries moves faster and sounds different from that flowing through normal vessels. TCD measures that sound and compares it to a normal reading to establish the exact configuration of the arteries in the brain.

People with sickle cell anemia or sickle cell trait are advised to avoid excessive physical exertion and exposure to high altitudes and excessive heat. Children with the disease who have had a stroke may need transfusions of normal red blood cells to prevent a second stroke.

Drug Abuse

Drug abuse is an ongoing national problem, particularly among young people. Stroke, both ischemic and hemorrhagic, is a common result of the use of a number of street drugs. There are several ways in which this can happen. Stimulants and hallucinogenics, including cocaine, LSD, and amphetamines ("speed"), affect blood pressure and blood vessels. Blood pressure races up when the drug is taken, partially because blood vessels narrow dramatically. This episode, called **vasoconstriction,** can prevent blood from continuing along an artery and supplying part of the brain with needed nutrients. An ischemic stroke results.

Drug users can also have strokes when they inject impure drugs directly into their bloodstreams. Some street drugs, including cocaine, are routinely "cut"—diluted with nonchemical binders—before they are sold and used for injection or inhaling. Drugs that originally come in pill form are sometimes crushed, mixed with water, and injected into the bloodstream. Fillers in the pills are thus injected along with the chemicals. These fillers can include diverse substances such as talc and cornstarch. The particles can travel through the bloodstream to the brain and cause embolic stroke when they finally block a small artery.

Cocaine and other stimulants can also alter blood and immune system functions. A blood clot may block the vessels, causing ischemic stroke, for example. When foreign substances are injected directly into the body, they immediately challenge the body's immune system, which swings into overdrive to get rid of the "invader." Eventually these extreme reactions damage both the immune functions and the arteries they involve. Stroke is especially likely for abusers who have been off a drug for a period of time and then suddenly go back on it. Their immune systems have had time to build up powerful antibodies to the drug. The antibodies overwhelm the system when the drug is reintroduced.

Hemorrhagic stroke is also a possibility for drug abusers, especially if they take stimulant drugs, or "uppers." Stimulants such as cocaine and speed raise blood pressure and blood flow very suddenly. Small arteries can rupture as a result—especially if aneurysms (weak spots in blood vessels) or abnormal arteries are involved.

Finally, the higher the dosage taken at one time, the more likely it is that the drug will trigger a stroke.

Tony was an energetic twenty-nine-year-old with many interests. By day, he was a computer programmer in a large corporation. On weekends he was outdoors, pursuing any of a number of favorite sports. He did everything from bicycling to tennis to basketball to swimming. He had a great body, and, hey, he liked to show it off!

Tony was socially active. Drugs, mainly cocaine, were frequently part of his socializing. Experimenting with drugs was just something his group did, and Tony never thought too much about it. He wasn't addicted. He said no to hits more often than he accepted them. But occasionally he took a hit when he was in a rowdy mood anyway. It never affected his health, and never would, Tony was sure. He was in top shape. Besides, he just wasn't the type to let drugs run his life.

One Friday, Tony received an unexpected promotion at work. He was in a great mood and thought he should celebrate. After work, he went running as usual. But this time he stopped about three miles into his route to look up his dealer and score a little cocaine for later in the evening.

His usual contact for the drug didn't seem to be around. Tony stood there for a moment, feeling a pinch of disappointment. Just a few moments later a man approached and struck up a conversation. The stranger, it turned out, had coke to deal himself. After a brief negotiation, Tony ran on.

He had invited some friends over that night to help him celebrate. Far into the evening, Tony offered them cocaine. Because it was his big night, Tony's friends insisted he go first. With a bit of a swagger and a deep breath, Tony inhaled a long line of the powdered drug through his nose. His friends hurrahed. Tony bowed.

Seconds later, Tony straightened up, a look of terrible pain across his face. And just as suddenly, he slumped unconscious to the floor. His friends could not get him to stir. They called for an ambulance, and Tony was rushed to the emergency room of the local hospital.

After what seemed like an eternity, Dr. Ling came out to talk to Tony's friends. She wanted details of their evening together and a sample of the drug Tony had taken. She told them Tony had experienced a stroke and she suspected the cocaine had triggered it.

Laboratory tests confirmed Dr. Ling's suspicions. The cocaine Tony bought was very pure. It hadn't been "cut" as much as his usual purchases were to dilute the stimulant effect. When Tony inhaled the drug through his nostrils, his blood pressure soared in response. Then his blood vessels constricted. An aneurysm—an existing weak spot along a major artery in his brain—hadn't been able to withstand such unnatural punishment, and it had burst. He had experienced a major hemorrhagic stroke.

The outlook for Tony's recovery, unfortunately, was poor.

The Stroke Risk Profile

Stroke is rarely attributable to just one cause. More often a variety of factors are at work. Thus a stroke risk assessment that is based on only one risk factor may needlessly alarm or falsely reassure someone. Multiple risk factors must be considered together in order to accurately evaluate a person's risk for stroke. Interestingly, one-third of all people who have a stroke share a certain combination of risk factors. These include systolic hypertension (high blood pressure), high serum cholesterol levels, diabetes, cigarette smoking, and an enlarged left ventricle of the heart. If you have all these factors, you should be closely monitored by your doctor. A "Stroke Risk Factor Prediction Chart and Worksheet" have been developed to enable doctors to accurately evaluate these and other risk factors. The chart and worksheet have been modified and combined in the "Stroke Risk Prediction Chart" on pages 80–81. You and your doctor can use this chart to put pieces of information together to come up with a composite risk profile for you.

The prediction chart considers nine conditions that especially affect stroke risk. Points are assigned to each condition depending on the presence, absence, or severity of the risk factor. The greatest risks are assigned the highest values. The final score indicates your likelihood of stroke within a ten-year period. The higher the total point value, the greater the risk of stroke. One part of the chart allows comparison between an individual's risk and the average risk for others who are the same age. Men and women are evaluated separately.

STROKE RISK PREDICTION CHART

1. IDENTIFY YOUR RISK FACTORS

WHAT IS YOUR AGE?

Your age	Points		Your age	Points
Under 57	0		72–74	6
57–59	1		75–77	7
60–62	2		78–80	8
63–65	3		81–83	9
66–68	4		84–86	10
69–71	5			

WHAT IS YOUR SYSTOLIC BLOOD PRESSURE?[1]

MEN		WOMEN			
Add 2 points if under treatment for hypertension		Not being treated for hypertension		Being treated for hypertension	
Pressure	**Points**	**Pressure**	**Points**	**Pressure**	**Points**
95–105	0	95–104	0	95–104	6
106–116	1	105–114	1	105–114	6
117–126	2	115–124	2	115–124	7
127–137	3	125–134	3	125–134	7
138–148	4	135–144	4	135–144	7
149–159	5	145–154	5	145–154	8
160–170	6	155–164	6	155–164	8
171–181	7	165–174	7	165–174	8
182–191	8	175–184	8	175–184	9
192–202	9	185–194	9	185–194	9
203–213	10	195–204	10	195–204	10

DO YOU HAVE A HISTORY OF DIABETES?

No	0 Points	Yes	2 Points (men)	3 Points (women)

ARE YOU A SMOKER?

No	0 Points	Yes	3 Points

DO YOU HAVE A HISTORY OF HEART OR BLOOD VESSEL DISEASE?[2]

No	0 Points	Yes	3 Points (men)	2 Points (women)

DO YOU HAVE ATRIAL FIBRILLATION?[3]

No	0 Points	Yes	4 Points (men)	6 Points (women)

DO YOU HAVE AN ENLARGED HEART?[4]

No	0 Points	Yes	6 Points (men)	4 Points (women)

2. ADD UP YOUR POINTS

AGE	HEART OR BLOOD VESSEL DISEASE
BLOOD PRESSURE	ATRIAL FIBRILLATION
DIABETES	ENLARGED HEART
SMOKER	

TOTAL POINTS

[1] Use systolic blood pressure, the higher of the two numbers in a blood-pressure reading (120 is the systolic pressure in a reading of 120 over 80, for example).

[2] Includes myocardial infarction (heart attack), angina (chest pain), coronary insufficiency (narrowing of the coronary blood vessels), intermittent claudication (narrowing of the arteries in the legs), and heart failure.

[3] Atrial fibrillation is a type of rapid, irregular heartbeat.

[4] Left ventricular hypertrophy, or enlargement of the heart's left ventricle. Reduces the heart's pumping ability, increases the risk of blood clots.

3. FIND YOUR STROKE RISK OVER THE NEXT 10 YEARS

MEN POINTS	RISK	WOMEN POINTS	RISK
1	2.6%	1	1.1%
2	3.0%	2	1.3%
3	3.5%	3	1.6%
4	4.0%	4	2.0%
5	4.7%	5	2.4%
6	5.4%	6	2.9%
7	6.3%	7	3.5%
8	7.3%	8	4.3%
9	8.4%	9	5.2%
10	9.7%	10	6.3%
11	11.2%	11	7.6%
12	12.9%	12	9.2%
13	14.8%	13	11.1%
14	17.0%	14	13.3%
15	19.5%	15	16.0%
16	22.4%	16	19.1%
17	25.5%	17	22.8%
18	29.0%	18	27.0%
19	32.9%	19	31.9%
20	37.1%	20	37.3%
21	41.7%	21	43.4%
22	46.6%	22	50.0%
23	51.8%	23	57.0%
24	57.3%	24	64.2%
25	62.8%	25	71.4%
26	68.4%	26	78.2%
27	73.8%	27	84.4%
28	79.0%		
29	83.7%		
30	87.9%		

4. COMPARE WITH THE RISK FOR THE AVERAGE PERSON YOUR AGE

MEN AGE	RISK	WOMEN AGE	RISK
55–59	5.9%	55–59	3.0%
60–64	7.8%	60–64	4.7%
65–69	11.0%	65–69	7.2%
70–74	13.7%	70–74	10.9%
75–79	18.0%	75–79	15.5%
80–84	22.3%	80–84	23.9%

This chart is based on one developed for the American Heart Association by researchers associated with the Framingham Heart Study. The original chart helps doctors create a composite stroke risk profile for their patients. Each patient can be evaluated on the presence, absence, or severity of several risk factors. These include sex, age, cardiovascular disease, and diabetes. This chart has been modified for easy use.

To determine the risk of stroke, the chart looks at the following conditions:

- sex
- age
- systolic blood pressure
- whether you are under treatment for hypertension (high blood pressure)
- your history of diabetes
- whether you smoke
- your history of heart or blood vessel disease
- your history of atrial fibrillation
- whether your heart's left ventricle is enlarged

(Atrial fibrillation is a condition in which the two upper chambers of the heart stop beating rhythmically and instead quiver ineffectively.) Completing the chart can give both you and your doctor a clearer idea of where to concentrate stroke prevention efforts if they are called for.

A kit containing the original "Stroke Risk Factor Prediction Chart and Worksheet" is available to physicians and other health care professionals through local American Heart Association offices. (Consult the list of AHA affiliates on pages 308–309 or your local telephone directory's white pages for the AHA office in your area.) A similar kit, focusing on coronary heart disease, is also available. Because heart disease is a risk factor for stroke, completing that worksheet might also be a good idea for those who are interested. The kits are based on data compiled from the more than 5,000 men and women who have been followed as part of the landmark Framingham Heart Study for more than forty years.

Francisco, seventy-five, had a number of stroke risk factors. Dr. Cohen used a "stroke risk prediction chart" to calculate Francisco's estimated risk of having a stroke. (Please look at the "Stroke Risk Prediction Chart" on pages 80–81 as we go.)

Dr. Cohen started with Francisco's age, which was assigned a value of 7 points. Next, he found his patient's systolic blood pressure level reading of 188. It was assigned a value of 8 points.

As a male diabetic, Francisco was assigned 2 points. He smoked; that was an additional 3 points. He had recently been diagnosed with angina pectoris, a heart condition, so his doctor added another 3 points to his score. The left ventricle of Francisco's heart was normal. Then the doctor added them all up.

Francisco's total came to 23 points ($7 + 8 + 2 + 3 + 3 = 23$). According to the chart, that meant that he had a 51.8 percent chance of having a stroke within the next ten years. That is more than a one-in-two chance of having a stroke, Dr. Cohen emphasized. Francisco was almost three times as likely as other men his age to have a stroke. (According to the chart, the average risk for a seventy-five-year-old man is 18 percent.)

Dr. Cohen recommended that Francisco cut out smoking. He also emphasized the need to take the blood pressure medication regularly. Dr. Cohen recalculated Francisco's stroke risk, using new figures to show Francisco how to make a difference.

"Francisco, by bringing down your systolic blood pressure to 140, you 'save' 4 points. And if you quit smoking, that would save you another 3 points. Overall, you save 7 points. Let's see, that lowers your point total to 16.

"According to the chart, a score of 16 brings down your stroke risk to 22.4 percent. That's roughly a one-in-five chance of having a stroke, and it's less than half the risk you carry now. It also brings you closer to the average risk of men your age."

By seeing his own risk factors personalized, Francisco was more easily convinced of the importance of quitting smoking and lowering his blood pressure. He resolved to work with Dr. Cohen and improve his health outlook.

The chart can be used by those with no history of cardiovascular disease as well as by stroke patients. It can give each person an idea of his own personal risk.

During a recent doctor visit, Ivy was interested in drawing up her own stroke risk profile. At age sixty, Ivy didn't smoke, wasn't diabetic, and had no history of heart problems. The left ventricle of her heart was normal. Her systolic blood pressure was about normal, at 123. She was not being treated for hypertension, or high blood pressure.

She and her doctor added up her points. Her age was worth 2 points. Her systolic blood pressure reading was assigned 2 points also. Otherwise, Ivy collected zero points from all the remaining risk areas.

With a total of only 4 points, Ivy had scant chance of having a stroke, her doctor said. The "Stroke Risk Prediction Chart" showed she had just a 2.0 percent chance of stroke within the next ten years. On average, in fact, others in Ivy's age group actually had more than twice the risk she did (4.7 percent).

Ivy's doctor recommended that Ivy continue to have regular medical checkups, keep an eye on her blood pressure, and watch her sodium intake as a further precaution.

What Does It All Mean?

People used to assume that good health was born, not made. You were lucky and healthy, or unlucky and unhealthy. And it's true, genetics do play an important role in determining the state of one's overall health. But it is increasingly clear that each individual makes choices in his life that can impair—or improve—that legacy. Every person can affect his own health for the better. Each individual can begin by eating sensibly, exercising regularly, staying away from detrimental habits such as cigarette smoking, and getting regular checkups. Identifying risk factors, and controlling or eliminating them, is also extremely important to achieving that goal.

But what happens if a stroke occurs anyway? Immediate emergency medical care is critical for the best outcome. In Chapter Three, we'll look at how a stroke is diagnosed at the hospital.

3
At the Hospital

DIAGNOSIS

Not so long ago, doctors could do little for the average stroke patient besides watch and wait until the condition stabilized. Today doctors have a better understanding of stroke. Doctors also have impressive resources available to help them give the best possible care to people who have had strokes. We are increasingly aware of how important it is for treatment to begin immediately. Doctors can limit the damage caused by stroke in some cases—provided treatment begins very soon after the stroke begins.

In this chapter, we'll look at stroke from the point of view of health-care providers. The world through the emergency room doors can appear very strange to those who aren't familiar with its fast-moving rhythms and special concerns. But as we'll see, every question a doctor asks and every test she orders is all part of an urgent effort to glean very specific information from the patient. Armed with that information, the doctor can accurately diagnose the patient's condition. Then she can begin appropriate medical treatment quickly and effectively.

Timeliness

Stroke, of course, is a medical emergency. Like any such emergency, it should be handled as a priority by all concerned. That attitude begins with the person who is having a stroke. Everyone should know the warning signs of stroke and be prepared to get medical help as soon as they are recognized. (Stroke warning signs are listed on page 37.)

Often these warning signs are relatively subtle, such as a weakness in a limb or a dimness of vision that passes after a time. It can be tempting to ignore the evidence of an impending stroke out of fear or a desire not to bother others over what appears to be a minor problem. Many people let several hours pass before heading for the hospital to check out their symptoms. Because in many cases they can still walk and talk, these people lack the sense of urgency that accompanies those who experience other medical emergencies, such as heart attack. Yet it is critical to understand that the earlier treatment begins, the better the chance doctors have to minimize permanent brain damage. How early is early? Some doctors believe that a person should get to a hospital within four hours after the stroke begins for early treatment to be most effective.

Luisa put down her paper and walked into her husband's study late one Saturday afternoon to ask him a question. But upon entering the room, she found her husband of forty-seven years struggling to rise from his chair. Hector had a panicky look in his eyes that told her something was seriously wrong.

It appeared Hector couldn't use his right leg or arm to help himself up. In addition, his efforts to tell his wife what he was experiencing were hard for her to understand; he seemed to have lost some control over speech, too.

A retired nurse, Luisa knew the signs of stroke when she saw them. She also knew from her newspaper reading that the hospital in their community had recently become involved in a stroke treatment trial. This treatment featured a new kind of drug. The news story had emphasized the importance of getting to the hospital as quickly as possible.

Reassuring Hector, Luisa went to the telephone and dialed 911. An emergency medical team responded quickly and got her husband to the hospital shortly after the stroke incident began.

Luisa waited while Hector underwent a number of tests, which she was told confirmed that Hector had had an ischemic stroke. After a little while, the attending emergency room doctor came out to speak with Luisa. The doctor brought a neurologist with her and introduced him to Luisa.

"Let me ask you something," the neurologist began. "We're conducting trials of a new drug, called t-PA, that has the potential to be helpful to some stroke patients who receive it. It is one of a class of drugs sometimes called 'clot-busters.' A blood clot caused your husband's stroke. This new drug may help dissolve such clots and restore blood flow to affected areas. Your husband has been selected randomly to participate in these trials if you give your permission. We think he is a good candidate because he got to the hospital so soon after the onset of his stroke. We must administer t-PA as soon as possible, however, if the drug is to benefit him.

"Before you decide, I must tell you that we don't yet know everything about this drug," the doctor cautioned. "We can't predict with complete accuracy how it will affect your husband, but obviously we think it may help him. There is, however, a small chance it will cause bleeding problems."

Luisa said she was aware that the trials were taking place. She asked the doctors a few questions before allowing her husband to participate.

Hector received t-PA soon thereafter. For him, the drug did what it was expected to do. His symptoms subsided, and he had what the doctors called "a good outcome." His only remaining difficulty was a mild weakness in one leg. Hector was able to go home with Luisa in a matter of weeks.

Initial Procedures in the Emergency Room

Timeliness is still vitally important once the person reaches the hospital. The attending doctor takes the patient's medical history, looking for risk factors and warning signs that may be lurking in the patient's background. Some of these might predispose the patient to either brain hemorrhage or ischemic stroke. Almost simultaneously, the doctor gives a complete medical exam as well as a bedside neurological exam. Depending on what he learns from each of these investigations, the doctor decides which tests to order to confirm or fine-tune the diagnosis. Once a diagnosis is made, treatment can begin. Some doctors believe a complete medical workup of this kind should be completed within an hour after the patient reaches the emergency room.

Routine Procedures

When someone who has had a stroke arrives at the hospital, some traditional emergency room procedures are followed as a matter of course. The patient's breathing will be checked to be sure that all airways are clear. His temperature and blood pressure will be taken. Other quick evaluations are done also. If he is dehydrated, an intravenous drip, called an IV, may be started in his arm to correct that problem. (Dehydration reduces blood volume and can potentially decrease blood flow through the body as well.) Usually the attending doctor will order routine blood and urine laboratory tests at this time.

Fifty-two-year-old Sudie grew very pale very suddenly one morning at breakfast. Her husband, Frank, noticed and asked what was wrong. Sudie whispered that she had developed a terrible headache and thought she would go lie down. Before she could, however, Sudie slumped over the table and lost consciousness.

Frank got her to the couch in the next room and then called immediately for an ambulance. At the hospital, Sudie was rushed into the emergency room, where she underwent a thorough workup. First her temperature was taken and her blood pressure was measured. Then blood tests were run and a urine sample taken. The attending doctor gave Sudie a physical examination and ordered a CT scan.

Frank called their daughter as soon as the hospital staff took charge of his wife. Grace arrived a short while later. Now they both felt they had been in the waiting room for some time without getting any closer to learning what was wrong with Sudie. What was taking so long?

When the doctor did appear, they were anxious to know what the delay had meant. Dr. Ivanoff explained that it was necessary to run a number of tests to determine the precise nature of Sudie's illness and how to proceed in treating it.

"We suspected a brain hemorrhage because of your wife's symptoms. The CT scan we ran just confirmed that," Dr. Ivanoff said gently. "Sudie has had a subarachnoid hemorrhage, which means a blood vessel has burst on the surface of her brain."

"You know, her mother had a stroke like that years ago," Frank told the doctor. "And so did her cousin. Isn't that strange?"

"Unfortunately, it isn't all that strange. It's not too uncommon for this kind of susceptibility to run in a family," Dr. Ivanoff said. "You did the right thing by getting your wife to the hospital so quickly. We're doing everything we can for her. Now let me get Dr. Carmine and introduce him to you. He's the neurosurgeon who has been assigned to this case. He should be just about finished interpreting your wife's test results so far. He'll want to explain to you where we go from here."

Blood and Urine Tests

Blood and urine analysis can alert the doctor to any chemical abnormalities or imbalances that might contribute to stroke. Any problems that are discovered may require follow-up tests. Younger patients at otherwise low risk of stroke may be screened for drugs of abuse as well.

A blood chemistry workup provides detailed information about a number of blood components. **Blood viscosity,** or thickness, affects how smoothly the blood flows through the vessels. A **blood hematocrit** count measures the number of cells in the patient's blood, which relates to how easily blood flows. **Fibrinogen,** a clotting component of blood, may also be measured.

Blood platelets, too, are counted. Platelets contribute to the blood's ability to clot over wounds and begin the healing process. When platelet counts are too high, unwanted clotting is more likely to occur. Low platelet counts may encourage bleeding. The time it takes for blood to clot, called the **prothrombin time,** is tested, too. This test is especially important for patients who are on certain anticoagulant (blood-thinning) medications or have a history of liver disease.

Stroke patients with high **blood sugar** or **calcium** levels tend to have a poorer prognosis than others. To help identify these patients, these components are looked at carefully. Finally, blood cholesterol levels may be checked. A high blood cholesterol level could suggest atherosclerosis and a thrombotic source of the stroke.

Although it isn't always possible at the time of the initial examination, a urine test is often ordered. It can help doctors reach a diagnosis in a couple of ways. Emboli sometimes travel to the kidneys as well as to the brain. Thus blood in the urine may indicate emboli as a cause of the stroke—as well as identify an additional problem for the doctor to take care of.

High Blood Pressure and Acute Stroke

Most stroke patients have normal or mildly elevated blood pressure when they arrive at the hospital. When high blood pressure accompanies stroke, doctors are very conservative in treating it during the acute stage. They bring it down very slowly, if at all. Bringing blood pressure down too rapidly, particularly in an ischemic patient, can further decrease blood flow. This situation can further damage the already blood-starved brain tissue affected by the stroke. Very high blood pressure is cautiously treated with fast-acting medication. If the blood pressure is not very high, the doctor will wait until the patient has stabilized before bringing it to within the normal range. Keeping blood pressure under control may help avoid another stroke.

The next step for the doctor is to narrow the initial diagnosis of "stroke" to one that is much more specific. She tries to identify the kind of stroke the patient has had (called **the stroke mechanism**) and to pinpoint precisely where it has occurred in the brain **(the stroke location).** These facts determine what the proper treatment will be. The physician's goals are to limit the extent of the brain injury, prevent complications from setting in as a result of the stroke, and stop the stroke from either progressing or recurring.

To do all that, however, first the physician must evaluate the patient and assess the patient's problem. She looks closely at the patient's physical and neurological symptoms. The doctor must also consider the patient's medical background and risk factors for stroke. All these taken together lead the physician to favor one diagnosis or another.

Patient History and the Physical Examination

The medical history and physical examination help the doctor determine what kind of stroke the patient has experienced. The doctor evaluates symptoms, looks closely at the patient's personal and family medical history, and examines the results of initial laboratory blood and urine tests. He will also want to know whether the patient has taken anticoagulants (blood-thinning medications) recently. The doctor will ask whether the patient has ever had a stroke before, and if so, what kind it was and where it was located in the brain.

In addition, the doctor considers the total medical profile of the patient. He looks at sex, race, age, and the presence or absence of medical conditions such as diabetes. All these factors affect the statistical probabilities of certain kinds of stroke affecting an individual patient. Detailed knowledge of individual risk factors helps the doctor create an initial hypothesis about the kind of stroke the patient has had and where in the brain it could be located. At the same time, the doctor starts to rule out unlikely sources of the patient's stroke. He will try to confirm or refute that educated hunch later, through additional tests.

As part of a complete physical examination, the doctor looks at the patient's heart, vascular system (the "waterworks" of the body, including the blood and arteries), and eyes.

Dan usually had a joke to share with everyone he met. But when doctors began examining him in the emergency room, it was clear he just wasn't up to it this day. He had drifted in and out of consciousness during the ambulance ride over.

Right now he could barely respond to doctors' questions, much less share his favorite jokes. Working quickly, the doctors examined him. They discovered a blood clot in one of the vessels in his right eye, which led them to suspect that Dan was having an embolic stroke. If they saw one embolism, there was a good chance there were others in his bloodstream, too. If one traveled up into his brain and got stuck there, it would block flow and cause the symptoms they were observing now.

"Run an EKG and a chest X ray, stat," the attending physician ordered. "Let's look at this gentleman's heart and see if it's behaving properly. And get Dr. Goldberg in here."

While the diagnostic tests were being concluded, Dr. Goldberg, a neurologist, conducted a bedside examination of the patient. Dan had roused a bit and was responding sluggishly to some questions. To an observer, the questions might seem almost insulting, they were so simple. But every question had a purpose. Each one could either eliminate a potential neurological problem or pinpoint one caused by the stroke. It was becoming increasingly clear that a stroke was what Dan had had.

"What were you doing when you started to feel bad, Dan?" Dr. Goldberg asked gently.

After a pause, the man responded weakly that he had been lifting a very heavy sack of dog food out of the back of his station wagon when it happened. The doctor noted Dan's response and continued to ask other questions that might shed light on the kind of stroke the man had had. In fact, many embolic strokes occur when susceptible people suddenly exert themselves. This information fit the pattern that was emerging from the doctor's other observations, such as that suspicious clot discovered in his patient's eye a short while before.

Dr. Goldberg pressed on, trying to determine what sort of neurological deficit might be involved as a result of the incident. He asked a number of disjointed questions in a row and noted the answers given or lack of comprehension shown by the patient. He was interrupted once, when Dan drifted out of consciousness briefly. He noted that, too, of course.

"Where were you born, sir?" the doctor asked. And, "Do you know where you are?" The questions kept coming, gently but firmly. "What number comes after seven, eight, nine in a series?" "Can you follow my finger with your eyes?" "Would you please cross out all the circles on this page with this pencil?" "Can you draw me a picture of a daisy?" Dan could answer some questions and follow some directions readily, but a few gave him trouble.

"Thank you, Dan," the doctor said finally. "You rest now. I'm going to check on your EKG and chest X ray, but I'll be back."

The EKG, a heart test, showed that Dan did have atrial fibrillation. With this condition, blood can pool and clot in some chambers of the heart. The clots can eventually be expelled into the bloodstream. There they either dissolve or travel until they reach a vessel so small they can go no further. If that happens to be a vessel in the brain, a stroke occurs. Blood can no longer be distributed through that vessel to the brain tissue, and it begins to die.

Sometimes, the clot can start to dissolve spontaneously, in which case the symptoms improve with time in the hours after the stroke initially occurs. Knowing this, Dr. Goldberg ordered an hourly repeat of the neurological tests he had given at his patient's bedside. Once he had an idea of how the stroke was progressing, he would go ahead with treatment for an embolic stroke, unless counterindications emerged in the meantime.

The Heart

The heart is routinely checked as part of many emergency room procedures. When stroke is suspected, however, the heart is given a much more thorough examination. Heart disease is a strong risk factor for stroke. A stroke may be the patient's first evidence of a heart condition; the two often go together. (For more information about the connection between heart disease and stroke, see Chapter Two.)

Because of this strong association, the doctor asks a lot of questions to try to get information about the patient's heart. He will also ask about possible evidence of prior transient ischemic attacks (TIAs). Has the patient had previous episodes of numbness or weakness in his limbs? When? Has he ever had visual problems or difficulty speaking that passed after a short while? When? If the patient had a TIA in the past, then his latest stroke is more likely to be of an ischemic origin, too. Because the patient is not always able to answer these questions for himself, a family member is often asked to recall any of the patient's similar incidents in the past.

The doctor will listen for heart rhythm disturbances, which can create emboli in the heart chambers. These emboli may travel to the brain, causing stroke. He will look for signs of congestive heart

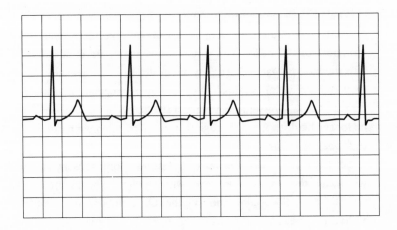

An electrocardiogram (EKG) produces a readout like this.

failure, which can affect the heart's ability to pump blood to all brain tissue adequately.

A chest X ray may be ordered, so the doctor can look for abnormalities in the heart's size. He may request an **electrocardiogram (EKG).** EKGs capture the rhythm of the heart as electrical impulses traced on a graph. This graph helps doctors evaluate the overall coordination of the heart muscle, as well as the spread of impulses through specific chambers of the heart.

The Vascular System

To identify blood vessel blockages that may have caused the stroke, the doctor checks the patient's vascular system carefully. He takes the patient's pulse at various places around the body, especially in the neck, listening for abnormal sounds or murmurs, called **bruits** (pronounced "broo-EE"). Comparing pulses taken from different spots like this helps the doctor zero in on just where the problem lies, if there is one. Such changes in sound can indicate the presence of atherosclerosis or diminished blood flow due to another reason.

The Eyes

Examining the patient's eyes is also important. In fact, some doctors consider the eyes a "window into the body's vascular system."

That is because blood vessels are easily observed in them, along with any evidence of vascular trouble. Patients who have had hemorrhagic strokes, for example, often show spots of blood in the tissues of their eyes. Other conditions affecting stroke—including high blood pressure, emboli, and ischemia—can leave their own evidence in the eyes. This, too, will contribute to the doctor's ultimate diagnosis.

Other Factors

While evaluating the stroke patient, the doctor must also pay close attention to conditions that may have prompted the patient to seek treatment. She will also ask questions about the onset of the stroke and the severity of the symptoms. She will ask about other symptoms that might have accompanied the primary symptom.

Hemiplegia, or total paralysis of one side of the body, is perhaps the classic sign of stroke. But not all stroke patients are hemiplegic. Many have hemiparesis, or partial paralysis of one side. Often the signs of stroke are much more subtle: numbness in the face, hand, or foot, for example. Problems with vision, speech, and balance are common. As the doctor examines the patient, she will check for headache, vomiting, and a decrease in the patient's consciousness level and ask when they were first noticed by the patient. (With subarachnoid hemorrhages, these conditions tend to appear abruptly. With intracerebral hemorrhage, they tend to appear later, while the patient's motor and sensory problems develop progressively.)

Headache can present special difficulties in the diagnosis of stroke. It is sometimes the only or primary symptom of hemorrhagic stroke. Many patients with subarachnoid hemorrhages who have a headache as the principal sign of the stroke show few other deficits or none at all. Because headache is such a common occurrence, it is important for doctors to try to get a very precise description of it. This description can come from the patient or, if the patient is unable to communicate, an observant family member. The best clues that the headache is associated with stroke have to do with its onset. The kind of headache most likely to accompany subarachnoid hemorrhage generally has an instant onset and is described by the patient as "the worst I ever had." Or the headache is accompanied at onset by a change in consciousness—fainting, convulsion, or collapse.

Like a reporter, the doctor will want to know "what, when, and where"—all the facts about how the stroke occurred. These help lead to a diagnosis. ("Why" the stroke happened, however, can't always be known for sure. This may be because available diagnostic techniques aren't yet sophisticated enough to identify every stroke mechanism, or it may be because some stroke mechanisms are still unknown.) The doctor is likely to "walk through" the onset of symptoms with the patient, if possible.

What was the patient doing when the stroke occurred? Although exceptions to the rule abound, thrombotic strokes very often occur at night or during a nap. Embolic or hemorrhagic strokes often occur when the circulation is more active, or when blood pressure rises. (Straining at a bowel movement or having sexual intercourse has also been known to trigger an embolic stroke.) But there is also plenty of evidence to show that thrombotic strokes can occur while the patient is active, and embolic or hemorrhagic stroke can occur when the patient is resting. These statistics are just that—statistics. They can contribute to the probability of a diagnosis, but they may not mean a lot to the individual patient.

The attending doctor will also ask the patient whether the main symptom (the weakness of the limb or inability to speak normally, etc.) seemed to improve or grow worse since he first noticed it. How the patient's problem develops can also give doctors a clue as to the nature of the stroke. **A problem that improves after onset** suggests a probable embolic origin of the stroke. The improvement may indicate that the embolism moved or dissolved, and blood was again able to reach the affected area of the brain.

A so-called **stuttering** or **stepwise onset** is one in which the patient's deficit improves and then worsens again one or more times. This sort of development may suggest a thrombotic origin of the stroke: Some blood is probably still able to pass through the partially blocked vessel. The third kind of stroke onset, in which the **onset of a problem is gradual** and accompanied by a headache, has been associated with intracerebral hemorrhage.

The Neurological Exam

While the physical examination helps determine the kind of stroke the patient has had, the neurological examination helps locate where the stroke occurred in the brain. This is possible because of the specialized way the brain is organized. Different functions are largely assigned to different areas of the brain (see illustration on page 12). To establish the kind and degree of neurologic disability the stroke caused, it is necessary to discover the patient's possible impairments in several areas. These include memory and language skills, behavior, alertness level, concentration, strength, muscle tone, orientation, vision and eye movement, and gait (the way the patient walks). Health-care professionals give the stroke patient a number of "spot tests" and gauge the results. For example, they might ask the patient where she is, a seemingly silly question that can measure her sense of orientation. Depending on the combination of impairments observed, the health-care professional can often estimate accurately where in the brain or neck arteries the stroke happened.

Stroke symptoms can develop over time, depending on the kind of stroke involved and its severity. Conditions can worsen before stabilizing. If this happens, physicians consider the stroke to be "progressing." For this reason, neurological tests, like physical examinations, are likely to be repeated for several days. After the first tests, a physician, nurse, or physician's assistant is likely to reexamine the patient at least every sixty minutes in the first hours after she is admitted to the hospital. Gradually this tapers off. Over the next eight hours, the patient will be checked every two hours. After that, she'll be checked at least once every four hours for new neurological deficits.

Language and Memory

The doctor, and perhaps a speech specialist as well, observes the patient to evaluate any language or speech difficulties resulting from the stroke. The manner in which the patient communicates after the stroke gives doctors some strong clues as to the stroke's location in the brain, as well as how best to proceed with rehabilitation efforts.

It's important first to distinguish speech from language. Language is the sounds, movements, gestures, and expressions we all use to communicate with one another. Speech is only a small part of language—the sounds we make with our mouths. Some people have trouble pronouncing words (a condition called **dysarthria**) but their language abilities are normal.

Speech and language problems can manifest themselves in many forms in stroke patients. (It may be helpful to review the discussion of the brain's cerebral cortex in Chapter One. That section outlines the areas in the right and left hemispheres that are largely responsible for the qualities and abilities that comprise human language and speech.) These difficulties fall into three general categories: articulating speech; understanding the spoken word; and reading and writing. A loss of ability in any of these areas is often due to **aphasia,** meaning "speechlessness."

Different Types of Aphasia

The term *aphasia* applies to a wide range of communication deficits. The ways we communicate with one another are very complex. An inability in even one area of communication can affect many other areas. Because of this, aphasias, too, are often very complex.

Some experts divide aphasias into three broad categories. In Wernicke's aphasia, the person is unable to understand language. In Broca's aphasia, the person has difficulty expressing himself. The third form of aphasia is called global aphasia. This is a combination of the other two types of aphasia. The person has difficulty both understanding language and expressing himself.

An overview of each of these is given below. For more complete information on a specif.c type of aphasia, ask the patient's neurologist.

Wernicke's aphasia. This aphasia is also known as sensory, receptive, or fluent aphasia. With Wernicke's aphasia, speech usually comes tumbling along in a steady stream, but doesn't make complete sense to listeners. Usually this person also seems to have trouble understanding what is said to him. He will also tend to make up words. The person with Wernicke's aphasia may not seem to notice that what he is saying isn't understood by anyone else.

Broca's aphasia. This kind of aphasia is also known as motor, nonfluent, or expressive aphasia. It makes speaking or writing difficult for the patient. Usually he knows what he wants to say and tries to make sense in his speech, but can't. Typically, he speaks in short bursts and repeats himself. Often he makes up words. Cursing is common. Because he is frustrated in getting out what he wants to say, the person with Broca's aphasia can easily become angry or depressed.

Others may have difficulty producing the names of people or objects—a condition called **anomic aphasia.** Some patients may also have related problems with reading and writing (called **alexia** and **agraphia,** respectively).

Simple oral and written tests gauge the type and extent of the patient's speech, language, and memory losses. Typically, the patient will be asked to repeat words and phrases, count, name objects, remember words, and follow the doctor's simple commands. He will be asked to read and write and to show he has understood what he has read and heard.

Dot had had a stroke several weeks ago, but today she was returning from the hospital to the apartment she had shared with her older sister Lois for seven years. Dot, a widow in her late sixties, and Lois, also a widow, lived in a retirement community. They both enjoyed participating in the activities offered there, from art classes to service projects.

Dot was looking forward to getting back into her old routine, but she was apprehensive, too. Her stroke had left her with a communication disorder that made it hard for people to understand what she said. She wondered how she would get along. Making people understand her could take so long now. And sometimes she found herself saying truly embarrassing things, without being able to control it. She was terribly worried that it might happen in front of her friends.

Lois, however, was completely excited. She had been looking forward to this homecoming for weeks and had planned a small reception in her sister's honor for that afternoon. "Bess, Phyllis, Ralph, and Pearl are stopping by later, Dot," Lois told her. "Don't worry, everything will be fine. They won't stay long. They're really looking forward to welcoming you home."

When the four arrived in the sisters' living room later that day, each one greeted Dot warmly. Lois ran back to the kitchen to bring out the refreshments. Dot wanted to thank them for coming and had many other things to tell them besides. But none of it was coming out right. When she tried, a stream of words came tumbling out, but they were just words without sense. The harder she tried to say what she wanted to say, the worse it got. She even swore a few times without meaning to.

Dot stopped in frustration when she saw the confused, surprised looks on her friends' faces. There was an awkward pause. Then Bess brightened and started to shout at Dot as though she were deaf. She thought that perhaps Dot wasn't responding intelligibly because she couldn't hear their comments properly. The others eagerly seized on that idea and began shouting at Dot, too.

Dot was thoroughly frustrated and angry now. She wanted to tell her guests that she could hear quite well, thank you, but she couldn't say that, either. It was bad enough to have had a stroke, but now she was being patronized, too! It was too much. She suddenly wished they would just go home and leave her alone. She felt very tired and stopped speaking altogether. She wondered what was taking Lois so long. Lois was always maddeningly slow, Dot thought.

At that moment, Lois did come back into the room, bearing a tray with cake and coffee cups and wearing a worried expression. She had heard the shouting from the kitchen and asked what was wrong.

"We're just talking with Dot," Phyllis said. "AREN'T WE, DOT?"

"Oh, dear," Lois said, setting down the tray. "You know, Dot can hear you clearly if you speak in a normal tone of voice. She's aphasic because of her stroke, but that's different from deafness. The kind of aphasia she has is called 'Broca's aphasia.' In fact, she not only hears you, but she also wants to respond. She just can't communicate what she wants to say very well because of the stroke. It can be discouraging for her, and I know it's new and frustrating for you, too. So please be patient, and please don't shout. Just listen carefully." Dot was relieved that her sister had spoken up, and she smiled encouragingly again.

Pearl, Ralph, Bess, and Phyllis apologized, but still looked a little uncertain about what to say next. Lois looked at her sister.

"Sis, you should slow down a bit when you talk, too," Lois reminded Dot as Lois began to cut the cake. Her eyes began to twinkle. "We all know how impatient you can be and how much you like to talk our ears off, but chill out, Sis. We've got lots of time! Cake, everyone?"

Behavior

Radical changes in a patient's behavior or personality after a stroke may also help indicate the location of the stroke. These changes can vary considerably. Some patients may become markedly apathetic to their environment. Others may do the opposite and become uninhibited and impulsive, showing inappropriate judgment in their behavior. These cases illustrate damage to the part of the cerebral cortex that controls complex behavior and some instinctual impulses.

People often rely on changing voice inflection and tone when communicating with others. But people with right-hemisphere strokes may lose this important component of human communication. Emotional tone, volume, and cadence in speech may disappear in these patients.

After a stroke, some patients seem unaware of their disabilities or are unconcerned about them, which complicates a treatment program. This condition, called **anosognosia** (pronounced "an-O-so-NO-zhe-ah"), is usually a result of brain damage in the right cerebral hemisphere.

Behavior is also affected if the inner, older part of the brain has been damaged by stroke. The limbic system, which is located underneath the cerebral cortex, controls our instinctual drives, including the "fight or flight" response, the survival instinct, and the sex drive. Strokes in this area, while much less common than those in the cerebral cortex, create an imbalance affecting instinctual drives. Some patients, for example, may become uncharacteristically aggressive or hypersexual. Some may become voracious eaters. Or the opposite of these problems could result, with patients losing normal interest in these activities.

Alertness Level

The patient's alertness level is important to assess. Decreased alertness—from drowsiness to unconsciousness—can be a sign of hemorrhagic stroke. It can also indicate a large injury affecting both cerebral hemispheres or an injury on the brain stem.

Vision and Eye Movement

The back of the brain is largely responsible for the interpretation of visual signals. When this area is damaged, it can cause isolated visual impairments. Stroke damage can affect vision on only one side or on both sides.

Stroke survivors commonly have visual field defects. This means they see only one half of the visual field the rest of us do when we use our eyes. Right hemiplegics tend to have trouble seeing to their right, while left hemiplegics have trouble seeing to their left. (You could get a sense of this impairment if you were to wear glasses affixed with black tape on the right or left half of each lens.)

Sometimes stroke causes damage in the nerve pathways to the brain that control eye movement. Usually strokes in the brain stem are responsible for this. Such damage may cause double vision or give a patient the feeling that objects in the field of vision are oscillating. The patient's eyes may be frozen to one side (known as **conjugate gaze paralysis**). They may oscillate, rapidly moving from side to side or up and down. Each of these possibilities suggests a different stroke site in the brain.

"Dad, you're wearing me out! I can't believe you've already had another fender bender. This is the third one in two weeks. What is going on with you?"

Reggie's son, Al, was exasperated and worried. His seventy-year-old father had indeed just been involved in his third minor accident in fourteen days. In all of the accidents, Reggie had bumped a car approaching from the right. It seemed more than a coincidence to Al, but his father refused to talk about it, brushing it off as a little bad luck.

"Your bad luck could kill you or somebody else, Dad. Maybe you should think about not driving. Jean and I would be happy to run errands with you," Al said.

"Humph," Reggie said. "I'm sound as a dollar." The two men were sitting in Reggie's cramped kitchen for this discussion. To change the subject, Reggie got up to get a snack from the refrigerator. He bumped into one of the kitchen chairs as he crossed the small room. Al noticed. That sort of clumsiness was becoming more pronounced, too. Could it be related to his father's driving problems?

The next day, Al called his father. "I'm coming by to take you in for a checkup with your doctor," Al said. Reggie protested, but Al insisted. "And don't worry, I'm driving," Al added cheerfully.

The checkup Reggie received was thorough. Back in the doctor's office, Reggie and Al met to discuss the doctor's findings. Dr. Rusk was able to diagnose that Al's father had had a small thrombotic stroke at the back of his brain. Using a small model of the brain to show father and son exactly what he was talking about, the doctor pointed to the area. This area was the visual cortex, he said. Reggie's stroke had damaged his brain's ability to interpret the visual cues it was receiving from the eyeball—but only half of it. Reggie could really see only half of everything in front and all that was to the left side of him. That was why he was bumping into things, large and small, that appeared on his right side.

"I'm going to start you on some medication that I want you to take faithfully," Dr. Rusk said, writing out a prescription. "It will help prevent any more clots from forming, and it may keep you from having another, more serious stroke in the future."

After discussing the medication with his patient for a bit longer, Dr. Rusk moved on to discuss Reggie's vision problem.

"You can learn to compensate for this deficit to a large extent," his doctor said. "You'll have to scan the area around you a bit more by turning your head from side to side, like this, but that way you should be able to see and avoid bumping most things.

"However," Dr. Rusk continued, "I'm afraid that driving is another matter completely. Your deficit creates a driving hazard to you and other drivers, as your accidents have proven. You simply may not drive any longer. I'm sorry."

"I don't want to hurt anybody, including me, of course," Reggie said. "But it will be hard to give up that license. And I really do feel fine."

"That's OK, Dad," Al said as they got up to leave. "We'll work it out. Jean and I really will be happy to drive you wherever you need to go. I mean that. It's just another way we can spend time together."

Gait

By watching the patient take a few steps around the room, the doctor can best compare the movements of one side of the body to another. She can detect subtle weaknesses that otherwise might easily be overlooked, such as a dragging foot or an arm that doesn't swing as much as the other. Incoordination or poor balance while walking might suggest a stroke has occurred in the cerebellum or brain stem.

The Motor and Sensory Systems

In addition to the tests described above, the doctor will evaluate the patient's **motor system,** or ability to move her limbs, after the stroke. He will extend the arm, shoulder, hand, fingers, leg, foot, and toes of the patient on both sides of the body. The doctor will test for strength, coordination, and reflexes in each area, then give the patient some simple tests that judge perception and other **sensory functions.** He may test perception by touching the patient's elbow and then asking her to close her eyes and touch the other elbow.

Noninvasive Tests

After the initial clinical examination, the attending doctor narrows the diagnosis of the patient's stroke to a few strong possibilities. Even different stroke patterns have many elements in common, however. For this reason, most doctors won't make a diagnosis on the basis of the patient's medical history and physical examination alone.

Now the physician confirms the diagnosis with some carefully selected laboratory tests. These tests are given sequentially. The results of each help determine what the next step will be. They give the doctor additional information about the stroke and also help determine ultimate treatment. The more common of these tests are discussed below.

Some of the best news recently in stroke care involves the development of noninvasive diagnostic techniques. As the term implies, these tests help doctors determine the type, location, and extent of a stroke without surgery or other invasive procedures. They provide accurate information quickly, safely, and painlessly. These techniques seek information about either of two conditions. Neuroimaging tests, such as CT scan and MRI, identify areas of tissue damage in the brain through pictures. Other new noninvasive tests examine blood flow and abnormalities of vessels in the neck and head.

Computed Tomography (CT)

Computed tomography, also called CT scan or cat scan, is an important basic neuroimaging test that evaluates brain tissue. It is usually one of the first tests scheduled for the stroke patient. The CT scan is a fast and painless way to determine immediately whether the stroke was due to bleeding (hemorrhage) or to a blockage (ischemia).

The answer to that question helps determine all further treatment. In a CT scan, the difference between bleeding and a blockage is as clear as black and white: A hemorrhage (bleeding) is identified by a white area, and an infarct (resulting from a blockage) by a black one. A CT scan can also rule out the possibility of a brain tumor as the source of the patient's problem. It can also uncover neurological injuries or brain abnormalities that the patient and doctor were not aware of.

A CT scan is most useful in identifying hemorrhagic stroke. It is extremely accurate in assessing the location and extent of damage caused by blood collecting in the subarachnoid space or within the brain substance. These areas show up in CT images as areas of higher density.

CT scans do have some limitations. They are not quite as precise a tool for learning more about ischemic strokes, although they can confirm the presence of one. Even large ischemic strokes don't show up for several hours. The test can miss small subarachnoid hemorrhages. Small infarcts, especially those in the brain stem, or lacunes deeper in the brain substance won't show up on a CT scan. Most TIAs aren't visible on a CT scan, either.

Magnetic Resonance Imaging (MRI)

This relatively new procedure uses a large magnetic field, which surrounds the patient's head like a halo, and radio waves to produce a three-dimensional, computer-generated image of the brain. (It can be used to image other parts of the body, too.) No radiation is involved. The patient must lie very still within the MRI scanner for thirty minutes to an hour while the image is generated. Because of the restraint this test requires, some patients find the procedure somewhat unpleasant. The doctor can help alleviate some of the anxiety with medication.

Both bleeding and blockages are easily identified by MRI. This diagnostic tool is especially useful for identifying blood vessel malformations.

MRI images give doctors a sharp image of the brain injury. Such clarity also means that they can pick up evidence of smaller injuries better than CT scans usually can. The test has advantages over CT scans in other ways, too. MRI is more capable of picking up strokes that occur in the back of the brain—in the brain stem or cerebellum, for example. It can also show small, deep strokes within the brain substance better than CT scans.

Where infarctions are concerned, MRI gives a clearer image of the damaged area than CT scans do. CT scans show the infarcted area as the same throughout. But in the early stages of ischemic stroke, infarctions are not the same throughout. The tissue at the center of the affected area is infarcted, or dead. For a little while, however, the rest of the area is still only ischemic, or dying. Theoretically it might be saved. (Sometimes this happens spontaneously, if collateral blood flow from neighboring arteries compensates quickly enough for the blocked blood vessels.) MRI can distinguish between infarcted and ischemic tissue. In the future, this capability may help doctors save ischemic tissue before it dies and therefore improve the patient's recovery outlook.

Magnetic Resonance Angiography (MRA)

Scientists are also trying to develop a procedure for using MRI to find evidence of atherosclerosis in the neck and brain arteries. If they are successful, MRI may someday replace conventional angiograms, an invasive procedure discussed on page 112. This new technique is called magnetic resonance angiography (MRA).

Like magnetic resonance imaging (MRI), MRA is completely noninvasive. Outwardly, the two technologies appear to be similar. Both utilize a strong magnetic field and radio waves interpreted by a computer to create a picture of the patient's brain. But MRA obtains quite different information for physicians.

MRA can create images of veins and arteries in both the neck and the brain. By creating a three-dimensional image of the information it collects, MRA is easier for doctors to use, too. Other tests show information in the form of graphs or two-dimensional pictures.

As this book is written (in 1993), MRA still has some limitations. For one thing, it is a very expensive technology, although costs are expected to drop as more people come to use it. The procedure is slow, too. To collect all the information needed to capture an image, the patient must lie very still under the MRA device for many minutes. That isn't easy for everyone to do. And not all vessels are shown clearly enough to be useful to doctors yet. But continuing improvements to this still very new technology are expected.

Ultrasound Testing

After a CT scan or MRI evaluation has been made, physicians may choose to run an individualized combination of ultrasound tests on the stroke patient, particularly if the stroke was ischemic.

Ultrasound is a noninvasive technique that helps doctors collect detailed information about the condition of some arteries. It is used most successfully on arteries located in the neck or at the base of the skull. Ultrasound testing can determine the extent and location of damage in these arteries. It can also collect valuable blood flow information pertaining to them.

To get an ultrasound reading, doctors place a sensitive probe over the suspect artery. This probe picks up information that goes back to a computer, where it is converted into images or curves on a graph. There are several kinds of ultrasound tests, as we will see next.

B-mode Imaging

This type of ultrasound testing is extremely accurate for evaluating the condition of the carotid arteries. An advantage to B-mode scanning is the fact that images can be established from several different planes, or levels, in the neck. This capability makes possible a detailed, three-dimensional image of the artery in question.

B-mode imaging shows doctors what kind of arterial injury they are dealing with. It also shows the severity of the damage. The test has its limitations, however. Blood clots may not show up, for example. Also, an artery that is severely narrowed due to atherosclerosis tends to look the same as one that is completely blocked.

Because of its limitations, B-mode scanning generally is used in conjunction with another ultrasound test, such as a pulsed Doppler test. The second test provides information that B-mode scanning cannot, such as blood flow velocities. Together the two types of ultrasound tests are called "duplex scanning." They round out each other's informational gaps and give a more complete picture of the condition of the artery.

Doppler Testing

In Doppler testing, as in other ultrasound techniques, a probe is placed on the skin over a neck artery. From this position it measures how fast blood is flowing through the artery. Knowing the speed, or velocity, of the blood can be very useful to doctors. From it, they can determine whether the artery is narrowed by plaque buildup and by how much.

How does that work? A blood vessel injured by atherosclerosis has a plaque buildup along its sides, somewhat like an accident on the side of the freeway. The plaque sticks out into the passage through which the blood flows, and in effect causes a backup on that freeway, forcing the blood to "merge" into fewer available lanes. This backup creates pressure behind the narrowed point. The blood that goes through the narrowed part of the vessel is consequently propelled past that point at a rate that is faster than normal. The change in blood flow speed at this point is what doctors measure. The greater the velocity of the blood flow, the narrower the blood vessel—and the greater the damage. Sometimes, however, no velocity measurement can be found. When that happens, doctors know that the vessel has been completely blocked and all blood flow has stopped.

Two types of Doppler tests are available that can take measurements of blood velocity in the neck. Continuous wave Doppler (CW Doppler) averages out the velocity of blood passing through a vessel beneath the probe to take a reading. The probe is moved along the neck above the course of the artery in question. Pulsed Doppler (PD) takes smaller, timed measurements over one spot in the artery to determine blood velocity.

If the doctor suspects that the patient has an atherosclerotic blockage in the arteries lying in the upper chest, above the heart but below the neck, other Doppler tests will be performed. Generally the blood velocities in each arm are measured and compared to determine any differences between them. Each arm is supplied with blood by the subclavian arteries, which give rise to the vertebral arterial system. Changes in the blood velocity in one of the arms tells doctors that there may be a blockage in either of these two arterial systems in the chest.

Color Doppler Flow Imaging (CDFI)

Color Doppler flow imaging is a new, more complete way to assess the condition of the neck arteries, especially the carotid arteries. CDFI gives doctors information about plaque composition in the arteries and blood flow velocity through them.

A two-dimensional image is created in color on a computer screen from the information picked up by CDFI probes. An advantage of this ultrasound method is that it creates immediate images of the arteries. Doctors consider these "real time" images superior to others because they are easier to see and interpret than the usual alternative—curves on a graph.

One drawback to CDFI is that doctors can't always make out the difference between an extremely narrowed artery, through which some blood still passes, and a completely blocked one. On the other hand, CDFI is very sensitive to finding even very small plaque formations in blood vessels in the neck.

Transcranial Doppler Ultrasound (TCD)

Unlike CT scans and MRI, transcranial Doppler ultrasound gives doctors useful information about the condition of the patient's intracranial blood vessels, rather than his brain tissue. Until recently, that information was only available through an invasive medical procedure called angiography (which will be discussed later in this chapter). TCD helps doctors precisely locate and determine the extent of atherosclerosis in the intracranial arteries. A microphone-like device is placed over strategic spots on the head. This device sends out ultrasound beams and picks up pressure and blood flow readings from the arteries at various depths. It then sends them back to a computer for interpretation. A complete workup takes approximately twenty to thirty minutes.

The principle behind TCD, as for all Doppler testing, is one that anyone who has ever been near a passing train has probably noticed. The sound of the approaching train changes as it comes nearer to you and changes again as it moves away from you. TCD picks up similar changes in the flow of blood through an artery. When an artery is narrowed, blood flow increases as a result of the smaller passageway. TCD can detect these changes and monitor them. If no signal at all is picked up, it tells doctors that the vessel may be completely blocked.

Duplex Scanning

Duplex scanning is a more complex form of ultrasound that also focuses on identifying vessel disease. It combines B-mode imaging with pulsed Doppler testing to give a more complete picture of atherosclerosis in the neck arteries than either test could provide by itself.

The pulsed Doppler test helps identify the arteries accurately and to orient the B-mode images correctly for interpretation. PD picks up evidence of blood flow changes in the arteries and evaluates the extent of that change. B-mode imaging helps doctors locate precisely where in the artery these changes are found.

Lumbar Puncture

This procedure is minimally invasive. Sometimes called a spinal tap, lumbar puncture gives doctors access to the brain's cerebrospinal fluid (CSF), the liquid that cushions the brain within the skull. A small amount of CSF is withdrawn through a needle placed in the lower spine. This is a routine, safe procedure that has been used by doctors to assess many kinds of neurological conditions, including stroke. Some patients have had headaches after the procedure. These go away within a few days. The procedure is a routine part of diagnostic evaluation in patients under forty with unusual symptoms.

Lumbar puncture can usually identify whether a stroke was hemorrhagic or ischemic. Blood or blood products in the CSF confirm a brain hemorrhage in most patients. Other abnormalities found in the cerebrospinal fluid may indicate an unusual cause of the stroke, such as meningitis. CSF abnormalities can also rule out stroke altogether, identifying a neurologic infection or inflammation that mimics stroke instead. Lumbar puncture gives doctors an accurate pressure reading of the body's central nervous system. In some cases, it is used to drain cerebrospinal fluid and relieve severe headache.

Lumbar puncture isn't appropriate for every stroke patient. In many cases today, CT scans and MRI can reveal much of the same information—without surgery—and are preferred where available. Noninvasive tests can usually identify intracranial bleeding, as well as the presence of tumors or other abnormalities with symptoms that mimic stroke. New monitoring devices can determine the patient's CSF pressure as well.

This procedure should be done only when other studies do not seem to give the necessary diagnostic information. Doctors avoid performing lumbar punctures on patients with intracranial hypertension or those with large hematomas, or pools of blood, in the brain. This is because of the danger of shifting brain position within the skull as a result of the difference in pressures above and below the brain.

Angiography

Noninvasive tests cannot always tell a physician everything he needs to know in order to diagnose a stroke accurately. Sometimes an invasive test—one that requires surgery or other invasive medical procedures—is necessary to complete the picture. Angiography is one such procedure that is commonly used to evaluate the size and location of blockages in the neck and intracranial blood vessels. This information is particularly useful if surgery is anticipated (such as carotid endarterectomy). (Arteriography refers to the same tests—called arteriograms—made exclusively on arteries.) Special dyes are injected through a tube into the blood vessels under investigation. These dyes illuminate or "tag" the vessels, as well as blockages, on X rays. Angiography can be especially useful in identifying bleeding aneurysms or arteriovenous malformations (AVMs).

Angiography is a standard means of evaluating the condition of blood vessels. (It can also be useful in evaluating coronary arteries.) Serious complications resulting from the procedure are infrequent and depend on a number of factors. These include the type of equipment and dye used, the amount of dye used, the number of injections made, the general medical and psychological health of the patient (i.e., the patient's attitude toward such medical procedures), and the experience of the angiographer. Traditional angiography may someday be replaced by a new technique called magnetic resonance angiography (MRA), which was discussed on page 107.

Complications

Stroke patients, like all other people who have had a major illness, are subject to complications arising from their condition. These tend to appear very soon after the stroke, and they should be anticipated by an alert medical staff. Following a stroke, patients may spend a few days in the intensive care unit (ICU) or special stroke unit of their hospital. In the ICU, their heart rates, brain functions, breathing, and other important functions can be monitored closely. Some of the major complications of stroke are infection, new thrombosis, paralysis, edema, seizures, and depression. These are discussed more fully on pages 131–137.

Conclusive Diagnosis

A thorough clinical examination coupled with individually tailored diagnostic tests gives doctors a great deal of information. In many cases, that is enough for the doctor to make a conclusive diagnosis. But that isn't possible in every case. Sometimes doctors never learn just how or why a stroke happened. Every doctor, however, should be able to confirm through examinations and tests whether the patient had a brain hemorrhage or an ischemic stroke. This basic information is crucial for determining appropriate treatment, which we'll discuss next.

4

Medical Treatment

A WAR FOUGHT ON MANY FRONTS

A s soon as doctors have diagnosed your stroke, they can begin treatment. That treatment has three main purposes: to stop further damage to brain tissue, to rehabilitate you, and to prevent another stroke. Ultimately, the goal of all treatment is to return you to the most independent life possible. The damage to the brain from stroke is permanent, but in many cases it can be compensated for to a large degree. In fact, many stroke survivors recover completely and return to fully independent lives.

Today stroke treatment can be individualized to each person's needs as never before. New therapies now under investigation promise even more beneficial treatment options in the future.

How does the doctor choose which stroke treatment is best for each individual? The stroke injury itself, which varies widely from person to person, is the doctor's most important guide. She must know where the stroke has occurred in the brain, its size, and the type of lesion (whether ischemic or hemorrhagic). If you have blood abnormalities or poor circulation, these related problems must also be addressed. At the same time, your doctor must take steps to lessen the chances of another stroke occurring and treat the medical complications that often accompany any serious illness.

Still other factors help determine your course of therapy. Your age alone rarely affects what your treatment will be. More important is your physical and mental condition apart from your stroke. For example:

- Major surgery to remove a leaky aneurysm might be fine for an older person in good health. But if you are the same age and also have advanced heart disease, this type of surgery may be unwise.
- Anticoagulant medication usually isn't the right answer if you are also severely hypertensive. The combination may increase your chance of brain hemorrhage.
- Someone with Alzheimer's disease may have trouble remembering to take medication every day as prescribed.

Each of these situations, and many others, can alter the nature of an individual stroke treatment program.

For many stroke survivors, rehabilitation training is also part of their regimen. That part of stroke treatment is discussed in Chapter Five.

Stroke hits people in one of two ways. Either the brain gets too little blood because of a blockage in the artery, causing an ischemic stroke, or an artery ruptures, causing a hemorrhagic stroke. These are two very different conditions, and they need different treatments.

Doctors can try two general approaches to improve blood flow to the area affected by ischemic stroke. One addresses the circulatory system and tries to improve the patient's overall blood flow, often by treating the heart and blood vessels. The other works by treating the blood itself, to prevent clots from forming and contributing to another blockage.

Improving Blood Flow

Often the quickest and most direct way to improve an ischemic stroke patient's circulation to the brain is simply to have him lie down. Placing the person in bed, with his feet slightly elevated, can help keep blood pressure levels up in normal ranges for those who are sensitive to a drop in blood pressure.

Blood flow through the arteries rises with increased blood pressure. For this reason, high blood pressure is generally tolerated during the early stages of ischemic stroke. If blood pressure is high enough to be life-threatening, the doctor will try to reduce it, but very slowly. If a patient's blood pressure drops too quickly, blood can't reach the circulatory system's outermost capillaries, in the same way a garden hose can't water the farthest corners of the garden if the water pressure drops suddenly. New brain damage to those areas could result. Similarly, fluid volume in the blood vessels contributes to the circulatory system's ability to keep blood moving strongly and steadily. If a patient is dehydrated for some reason and his blood volume is low, the doctor will correct the problem promptly.

Each of these methods attempts to improve blood flow by fine-tuning the mechanics of the circulatory system. But in some cases, doctors have another option as well. They may choose to surgically remove blockages from the artery instead. The most common procedure of this type is called a **carotid endarterectomy.** This procedure is performed on some patients who have had ischemic stroke or TIAs.

Carotid Endarterectomy

Carotid endarterectomy is a surgical procedure to treat atherosclerotic damage to carotid arteries, which run up along the front of the neck.

The two carotid arteries are among the four main channels by which blood is moved from the heart to the brain. The neck is a common site for this type of operation because the carotid artery branches here just before going into the brain. The extra turbulence generated at this fork in the bloodstream makes the area more susceptible to injury—and subsequent plaque buildup. Fortunately, the area is easily accessible to surgery.

Atherosclerosis has the dubious distinction of being the most frequent cause of stroke. It is a condition in which the artery's inner walls are damaged, sometimes exposing the tissue underneath. At the site of the damage, blood cholesterol, calcium, and blood components collect. Blood cells called platelets, which promote clotting, also pool there as part of the process. But because the platelets are sticky *and* stick out into the bloodstream, other materials from

the blood flowing by pile up and collect on them, forming **plaque.**
Plaque has two important effects. It causes more turbulence and
injury to the blood vessel underneath, causing more plaque buildup
and blockage. It also attracts more blood platelets to the scene and
creates blood clots. A clot that is attached to the plaque is called a
thrombus. A clot that detaches and travels farther along the bloodstream before getting stuck in a narrower channel is called an
embolus (plural: emboli). In either case, if the clot blocks blood
from continuing through the bloodstream, it can cause an ischemic
stroke.

The goal of carotid endarterectomy is to prevent an ischemic
stroke from occurring in the part of the brain served by the affected
artery. In this operation, part of the carotid artery's inner lining is
scraped away to remove the plaques that have formed there.

Carotid endarterectomy is a major surgical procedure, and its
risks must be evaluated carefully.

- The surgery is not appropriate for every person with
  diseased carotid arteries. The best candidates are those
  who have either had a mild ischemic stroke or shown
  symptoms of one in the form of a transient ischemic
  attack, or TIA.
- The surgery may not be appropriate for those who
  have artery disease but do not show symptoms. For
  them, the risks of surgery may be comparable to their
  risk of stroke. Studies are now being done to determine
  whether medical or surgical treatment is better for
  these individuals.
- The amount of blockage to blood flow in the artery
  itself is another important qualification for the procedure. The surgery is most successful when blood flow
  through the artery is at least 70 percent narrowed, but
  not completely blocked. If the artery is completely
  blocked, it cannot be reopened. Noninvasive tests,
  such as ultrasound, give doctors an accurate idea of
  the degree to which the vessel is obstructed.
- Finally, the person must be considered a "good surgical
  risk." That means he must be expected to recover from
  the normal rigors of major surgery and otherwise be

well enough to benefit measurably from the procedure. The person's life expectancy without the surgery must also be considered. Some people have specific conditions that would preclude this type of surgery, including: uncontrolled diabetes or high blood pressure; advanced cancer; a cardiac condition that may be the real source of the person's ischemic symptoms; or stroke symptoms of uncertain cause not related to the carotid artery.

The most serious risks of carotid endarterectomy are cerebral infarction and heart attack. Either of these can be life-threatening. Another serious risk, though uncommon, is the possibility of brain hemorrhage during surgery. Unblocking the affected artery occasionally releases a surge of blood into the region of the brain it supplies. This can overwhelm the already-damaged smaller arteries and capillaries along its route. High blood pressure increases the chance of hemorrhage, and blood pressure can go up after carotid surgery. For this reason, the patient's blood pressure is carefully watched and controlled after each surgery.

Proper scheduling of the operation can help avoid the possibility of hemorrhage, too. If you have had a large ischemic stroke, your brain should be allowed to recover before surgery. The surgery may be delayed as long as six weeks after the stroke.

Once your physician has decided which procedure is right for you, there is even more to consider. Some studies have shown that the success of carotid endarterectomy seems to depend greatly on the experience of the surgeon, anesthesiologist, and radiologist involved in the operation. It also seems to depend on the expertise of the hospital medical staff where the surgery is performed. Be sure to discuss these issues with your family doctor.

Carotid endarterectomy is an expensive procedure that has become increasingly common in this country since the early 1970s. Sometimes, however, outcomes are no better for the patient than the best nonsurgical care. Ultimately, there is much to consider before undergoing this procedure. Its value should be considered on a patient-by-patient basis. It should never be relied on to replace other medical measures or careful attention to the patient's other risk factors for stroke.

Abdul, sixty-five, was in his doctor's office, looking worried. He'd always had excellent health, he was telling Dr. Minton, but in the past month and a half he'd had episodes in which he felt weak, had blurry vision, and couldn't speak. They'd all gone away, but the last time it happened, yesterday, it had felt differ-ent—worse. The symptoms had lasted longer and he decided he'd better investigate it.

After examining Abdul, Dr. Minton told his patient that he was having transient ischemic attacks, or mini-strokes, and that they were indeed very serious. It was quite possible that they indicated a much larger stroke ahead, unless steps were taken. Dr. Minton wanted to run some tests and find out what might be causing these TIAs. Then he could make some suggestions about stroke prevention. He and Abdul would have to work together.

In the hospital, Abdul underwent a series of tests. One test revealed that his left carotid artery—one of four major arteries carrying blood to the brain—was 90 percent blocked with atherosclerotic deposits. There was no denying now that Abdul was at very serious risk of having a major ischemic stroke.

Because Abdul was in otherwise good physical condition and therefore a good surgical risk, Dr. Minton thought that a surgi-cal procedure to clean out that artery would be the best way to treat this particular patient. "You've already had these TIAs, so we know you're at greater risk of having a full-blown stroke than others who may also have a blocked carotid artery," Dr. Minton told his patient. "That makes you a stronger candidate for carotid endarterectomy right there. In this procedure, we scrape away the plaque that has built up along that artery, improving the blood flow to the brain," he explained. "It's a good idea to get rid of that plaque if we can—and we can, in your case. The deposits eventually can choke off all blood flow along that artery. Also, little bits of the deposit tend to flake off, creating emboli. And emboli can cause stroke in their own right."

Abdul agreed to surgery, which was performed successfully by a surgeon who specialized in the procedure. When Abdul saw Dr. Minton for his final postoperative checkup a few months later, Abdul said he hadn't had another TIA, "not even once," and was feeling as good as ever.

Angioplasty

In this procedure, a tiny device, typically a balloon, is slipped flat into the blocked blood vessel. It is then expanded to pry open the passage and restore blood flow. Angioplasty has already proven effective for heart problems. But it is still experimental and extremely risky where the brain is concerned. Angioplasty may become a viable means of treating ischemic stroke symptoms in the future. Before then, however, the technology will have to improve so that debris released during the stretching of the artery can be contained.

Treating the Blood

The other major means by which doctors can try to improve blood flow to the brain and prevent further ischemic problems is to treat the blood itself. The goal of this strategy is to maintain or increase blood flow by preventing thrombotic or embolic clots from forming.

Blood clots largely result from any of three problems:

- Imbalances in an individual's blood chemistry that cause an increased likelihood of clotting.
- Weakened or otherwise inefficient pumping action by the heart that creates pools of stagnated blood in the heart chambers. Embolic clots can form in these pools. The clots can then be pumped out of the heart and along the arteries to the brain (or other sites in the body, such as the lungs).
- Clotting by certain blood components at sites of atherosclerotic plaques. Clots form over the plaques and may either break loose and go to the brain or totally block the artery.

Each type of problem suggests a different therapeutic remedy.

Increased Tendency for Clotting

This informal term covers different disorders. One typical disorder is **polycythemia,** in which the blood produces too many red corpuscles. Another is **thrombocytosis,** in which the blood produces too many clot-forming platelets. Too much of the blood component **fibrinogen,** a clotting agent, can also cause problems.

If you've had a stroke, you will have a blood chemistry workup as soon as you are admitted to the hospital. This tells doctors immediately whether changes in clotting factors may have contributed to the stroke. Doctors may then treat the condition medically to obtain an immediate effect. You may be treated with a class of drugs called blood platelet antiaggregants. They work by preventing blood platelets from sticking together. They are discussed more fully on pages 122–125. Over the long term, however, doctors may choose to address the problem in nonmedical ways.

Clotting Associated with Heart Problems and Blood Stagnation

As many as 15 percent of all strokes are traced to emboli generated from the heart. Several kinds of heart problems can create emboli. By far the most common one is **atrial fibrillation,** in which the upper two chambers of the heart beat rapidly and ineffectively instead of strongly and efficiently. This condition allows blood to pool in those chambers, which can allow emboli to develop. Nearly 2 million Americans have atrial fibrillation. **Myocardial infarction,** or heart attack, kills some of the heart muscle, which reduces the heart's ability to beat as strongly as before. This may allow emboli to form in some heart chambers. Blood clots can also form around heart structures damaged by **rheumatic heart disease** and around **artificial heart valves.**

To treat clotting, doctors rely on a medical therapy of anticoagulants, or "blood thinners," which can make it harder for clots to form. The outcome of anticoagulant treatment can vary, depending upon the heart condition causing the emboli. Most evidence shows that this type of therapy helps prevent recurrent embolic stroke in the heart.

The use of anticoagulants is not without risk. Before administering them, doctors will perform tests such as CT scan and lumbar puncture to be sure a hemorrhage has not occurred. Even after these precautions are met, however, certain risks remain. One of them is hemorrhage, especially brain hemorrhage. That risk is generally small *unless* the patient has very high blood pressure *and* has had a large cerebral infarct recently, is prone to falls, or abuses alcohol. The patient must be especially careful to avoid any new injuries while taking anticoagulants, because it may be hard to stop any bleeding that results.

Ultimately, the doctor must decide what is best for the particular patient. He must determine whether the patient's risk of further embolic stroke without the therapy outweighs the risk of brain hemorrhage with it.

Anticoagulants are complex drugs. Treatment should be carefully supervised, and it should last only as long as necessary. Anticoagulant medication comes in two basic forms, heparin and warfarin.

Heparin

This natural substance prevents blood from clotting. Heparin must be given by injection, and it is usually given at the hospital. When it is given intravenously, it acts immediately. Although not of proven value, many doctors use heparin during the acute stroke stage hoping to prevent further clot formation. Sometimes it is administered to prevent clotting at the site of a very tight stenosis, or blockage, of a large artery. Patients do not stay on heparin indefinitely; the typical therapy with this drug lasts a few days.

Warfarin

Warfarin works as an anticoagulant by preventing some blood clotting agents from forming in the liver. Warfarin therapy often is given along with heparin at first. Warfarin takes several days to be fully effective. It is taken in pill form, and it is designed for long-term use.

Clotting Associated with Injury to the Blood Vessel

Atherosclerosis, as mentioned earlier, is the process by which damage to the blood vessels can stimulate the formation of clots. **Blood platelet antiaggregants** can prevent clots from forming. They do so by preventing blood platelets from sticking together to start the clotting process. They are used as a treatment for patients with atherosclerosis or those with increased clotting tendencies. Platelet antiaggregants are also called **platelet inhibitors.** They are generally prescribed preventively, when atherosclerosis is evident but there is not yet a large obstruction in the artery. Blood platelet antiaggregant drugs include aspirin, ticlopidine, and dipyridamole. Of these, aspirin and ticlopidine are the most commonly used.

Aspirin
Right now, aspirin is perhaps the single most important therapeutic agent for stroke prevention. Some studies have shown that taking four adult tablets a day reduces the chance of stroke by approximately 25 to 30 percent.

Studies are being done to investigate the possible effects of long-term aspirin use, including the risk of gastrointestinal side effects. One question yet to be answered definitively is the optimal daily adult dosage of the drug for the purpose of stroke prevention. For now, your doctor may recommend you take between one and four adult tablets every day, depending on your medical condition. If you don't tolerate aspirin well, you should take only the minimal dosage recommended by your doctor.

Aspirin is inexpensive, generally safe, and well tolerated by most

---

TRADE VS. GENERIC NAMES
OF SOME COMMON STROKE MEDICATIONS

Hearing some doctors talk about medications can really try your patience. While physicians swing easily between the trade and generic names of the medications they discuss, they sometimes forget to translate these terms for their listeners.

Generic Name	Trade Name
heparin	Heparin
warfarin	Coumadin®
aspirin	sold under several trade names in several different preparations
ticlopidine	Ticlid®
dipyridamole	Persantine®

people. But this common compound is anything but simple. Because it is so familiar, many of us take it without thinking of possible side effects. Like any other drug, however, it has some, such as gastric discomfort and gastric ulcers. Aspirin triggers a number of complex biochemical reactions in the body. Some of them help stroke patients by inhibiting blood platelets from sticking together. But other effects are less well understood. For this reason, you should never take aspirin over a prolonged period without checking with your doctor first. He will recommend an appropriate dosage, which you should take only under his continuing supervision.

Aspirin therapy can't "cure" atherosclerosis—it simply reduces some of its consequences. People with evidence of atherosclerosis can eliminate or reduce many of the risk factors that can contribute to the formation of new plaques. (Risk factors are discussed in Chapter Two.) As a further precaution, however, doctors often keep patients on aspirin therapy indefinitely, once it is begun.

Several years ago, Max, a retired postal worker, had been diagnosed with high blood pressure. He had been given medication to help bring it down to a normal range. Oh, he had taken it faithfully for a long time. But he'd be the first to tell you that he eventually grew tired of that routine. Such a bother. He'd felt fine, so it couldn't be that important, right? He would add that this attitude drove his wife, Emma, crazy. She loved doctors, but he sure didn't. When Emma mentioned his medication, Max would laugh charmingly and throw his hands up in the air as if to say, "That's just the way I am!"

A few months ago, however, Max had had a mild stroke, rebounding fairly quickly. Tests did not uncover evidence of carotid artery disease, an elevated platelet count, or any other obvious cause of his stroke. His doctor decided that, to be on the safe side, he would put Max on aspirin therapy, to reduce further stroke risk.

"But I plan to monitor you closely, Max," his doctor warned him. "I want you to take the aspirin exactly as I prescribe it, and I want you to keep your blood pressure under control, too. I don't want to hear that you've been careless about this course of therapy. It is very important to keep your blood pressure under control."

Max was smiling, but looked noncommittally at his physician. Next to him, Emma rolled her eyes and shook her head ruefully. The doctor took a deep breath and decided to unload the big guns. "You should know, Max, that I've made your wife my unofficial deputy in this. She has my permission to hound you about it whenever you forget to take your aspirin or your blood pressure medicine. You must take your medication— exactly as prescribed. Now do we have a deal?"

Emma cheered. She turned to her husband and said impishly, "I could enjoy that, you know."

Max decided he knew when he was surrounded. He laughed and shrugged. "I can't lose with all this attention! I'll take care of it, doctor, just as you say. Because I know that otherwise, Emma here will take care of me!"

Ticlopidine

Ticlopidine is a new drug that may prove to be more effective than aspirin in preventing further stroke after TIA or stroke. It is also more expensive than aspirin. Like aspirin, ticlopidine helps prevent clotting by keeping blood platelets from sticking together. It is known to be equally beneficial for men and women.

Ticlopidine therapy, like aspirin therapy, does carry some risk of side effects. Most are not serious enough to warrant suspending treatment, however. Gastrointestinal problems, especially diarrhea, are the most common side effect. Skin rash is another. Ticlopidine's most serious known potential complication is that it may reduce the body's number of infection-fighting white blood cells. This condition, called **neutropenia,** occurs in about 1 percent of patients who receive the medication. These patients can be identified with blood monitoring during the first three months of ticlopidine therapy. If the condition occurs, it is reversible. Those who can't tolerate ticlopidine for any of these reasons are likely to go on some form of aspirin therapy instead.

A New Idea in Stroke Treatment

Thrombolytic agents are experimental drugs that may prove beneficial to ischemic stroke patients in the future. One of them is tissue plasminogen activator (t-PA), nicknamed a "clot buster." This compound is the modern product of gene-splicing. It works by dissolving blood clots in arteries going to the brain, thereby relieving ischemic symptoms. Many heart patients benefit from thrombolytic agents. Studies are now under way to determine if these drugs will benefit stroke patients as well.

Doctors already know that thrombolytic agents are not beneficial to stroke patients if the medication is administered too late after the stroke begins—perhaps after an hour or so. (The exact window of opportunity is still under investigation.) Clearly, if these drugs become an accepted treatment for stroke, only people who recognize their symptoms and get to a hospital quickly will benefit.

Theoretically, this noninvasive method of eliminating blockages in blood vessels may be of great value. But these powerful drugs also carry an increased risk of brain hemorrhage. These risks will have to be investigated and carefully evaluated before thrombolytic agents become a treatment for stroke.

Treating Hemorrhagic Stroke

Ischemic stroke, as we have seen, requires attention to restoring or improving circulation to the brain. Hemorrhagic stroke requires a different approach. The goal in this case is to limit the damage the hemorrhage causes. One way to do this is to bring the patient's high blood pressure into the normal range. The doctor may also treat any swelling and drain blood from the brain, if necessary. She may also surgically remove arteriovenous malformations (AVMs) or treat aneurysms, weak spots in blood vessels, that are the source of hemorrhage. (AVMs and aneurysms are discussed on page 128.)

Control High Blood Pressure

Most intracerebral hemorrhage in people who don't have aneurysms or AVMs is due to high blood pressure. So, using drugs that bring down high blood pressure is important in these cases. But it can be a complicated procedure immediately after a stroke, and it must be done very slowly and conservatively. Moderately elevated blood pressure immediately following a stroke is actually helpful. It keeps blood flowing to the outermost capillaries of the nearby cerebral arteries that have not been affected. These capillaries normally overlap a bit with those from other arterial systems to ensure that all parts of the brain are supplied constantly with blood. During a stroke, like good neighbors, the intact capillaries continue to provide blood to some of the affected tissue. If the patient's blood pressure is brought down too quickly, however, blood won't be able to reach those outermost capillaries, and the brain tissue can die.

Treat Swelling

Brain swelling can follow a large ischemic stroke or an intracerebral hemorrhage, generally within four days. This serious and fairly common complication doesn't affect every person who has a stroke. The greater the swelling, or edema, the worse the prognosis.

Symptoms of edema may include a bad headache, difficulty walking, nausea, and vomiting. The person's consciousness level is also affected and is a sign of the edema's severity. A person with brain edema may experience drowsiness that comes and goes or lapse into unconsciousness altogether. Because edema can be caused by several different conditions resulting from stroke, treatment varies. A number of drugs can effectively reduce edema.

Drain Hematomas

Hematomas are local pools of blood sometimes found in the brain after hemorrhage. In the skull, where there is little extra space to spare, a hematoma can dangerously increase pressure on the brain, causing further injury. It is sometimes necessary to drain the hematoma to relieve that pressure. This is done if the hematoma is life-threatening and if it is in a place accessible to surgery. Sometimes hematomas drain spontaneously into the brain's subarachnoid space or into one of its ventricles, or cavities. From there, the fluid is reabsorbed slowly into the body.

Hematomas can cause periods of unconsciousness. Patients with very large hematomas over their dominant cerebral hemisphere have a smaller chance of recovery. For them, neither surgery nor medication is likely to be of much help.

Remove Aneurysms or AVMs Surgically

Most aneurysms are related to artery wall defects that were present at birth. Over a lifetime, these weak spots in the blood vessels tend to become thinner and balloon out. The thinner they get, the more likely they are to leak or rupture. That causes severe, immediate headache as the escaped blood pools and exerts pressure in the closed quarters of the skull.

Surgery often is called for if an aneurysm or arteriovenous malformation (AVM) leaks. After an aneurysm leaks once, it is quite likely to leak again, usually within two to three weeks after the first event. Or it may rupture entirely, resulting in a full-blown stroke. So far, surgical treatment generally is not recommended for aneurysms that do not already show signs of leakage.

Other Measures

When treating a patient with hemorrhagic stroke, physicians also treat special blood problems or conditions that might contribute to the patient's blood loss. For example, if the patient experiences bleeding because of ongoing anticoagulant therapy, his therapy must be revised. If the patient has hemophilia or other tendencies for bleeding, they can be treated also.

Ken worked hard, typically long days as a broker for a major securities firm in a large city. He thrived on adrenaline; he lived for making deals.

When Ken wasn't working, he was rock climbing or running, often with his girlfriend, Jennifer, who was also athletic. Ken was in good shape, except for a high blood pressure condition his doctor had detected in a routine checkup. It was high enough for the doctor to prescribe medication, but Ken was erratic about taking the drug. It made him feel silly to take it, as though he were sick. And anyone could see he was in the pink of health. He felt great!

He was having his usual bagel and coffee at his desk early one morning when he was overcome by a headache unlike any he had ever felt before. It made him nauseated; he felt as though his head would explode. Coworkers at adjacent desks had just noticed that Ken was behaving oddly and moving much more slowly than usual. Suddenly Ken slid to the floor and lost consciousness. "Someone call an ambulance!" was the last thing Ken heard.

At the emergency room, doctors huddled around Ken's CT scan. "There it is," said one, pointing to a white area clouding the computer-generated picture of Ken's brain tissue. "That's where the hemorrhage is."

Another doctor agreed. "Looks like a ruptured aneurysm, all right."

Taking into account Ken's age and general health, which was good, the doctors recommended to Ken's family that it would be prudent to operate and try to repair the broken blood vessel. They agreed. The neurosurgeon came over to talk to them about the surgery.

Jennifer, who had come to the hospital, too, listened carefully. She then spoke up with a question that had been bothering her.

"I know Ken hasn't been taking his high blood pressure medication. Are you going to bring down his blood pressure before you operate?" she asked. "Isn't it dangerous to let it go any longer?"

The attending physician shook his head. "Actually, if we were to bring down his high blood pressure too suddenly right now, Jennifer, we could cause more damage to Ken's brain tissue. Moderately high blood pressure temporarily helps preserve some of the injured brain tissue after a stroke like this. We will monitor it, though, and bring it down slowly and conservatively at the right time. Try not to worry. We're going to do everything we can for Ken."

In the Future:
Helping the Brain Survive Stroke

Traditional stroke treatment has always focused on what can be done for a patient *after* the acute stroke episode is over. But as scientists continue to unlock the secrets of brain function, they are also establishing new, experimental approaches to stroke treatment. By studying the chemistry of the brain, they are learning better ways in which to intervene and protect the brain cells during the actual stroke. If they are successful, they may be able to save brain tissue in the future that is lost to stroke today.

The key to this approach is to interrupt the chemical chain of events that leads to permanent brain damage *as it happens.* Timing will be critical. It will be even more important than it is now for a person who is having a stroke to get to the hospital immediately. People often recognize the need to get prompt medical care at the first sign of heart attack. This kind of thinking is only now becoming widely accepted for stroke.

By investigating brain cell function, scientists have learned that it may be possible to intervene medically during a stroke to protect some brain tissue. During ischemic stroke, one central area, served mainly by the blocked artery, quickly starves to death for lack of blood, causing an infarction. But a secondary, outlying area that is also affected by the stroke goes through an intermediate stage before suffering the same fate. This is the area that doctors hope someday to be able to save. The brain tissue in that outlying area hangs on by getting some nourishment from neighboring, unaffected blood vessels. (Adequate blood pressure actually helps here. Behind a blocked artery, blood pressure drops. This vacuum "encourages" blood from other areas to rush in and reestablish a stable pressure.)

For a short time, that tissue hovers between life and death. In boxing terms, it is down, but not yet out. Technically, doctors say that tissue is ischemic, or starving and stunned. If the blood supply isn't reestablished rapidly, certain chemical imbalances result. This in turn trips adverse reactions in the brain cells. These reactions, scientists suspect, are really responsible for the death of the brain tissue. By somehow interrupting those chemical reactions, they hope to learn how to buy time—time to restore blood flow to the ischemic area before it dies. Doing so could save brain cells—and precious brain function.

Brain temperature has also been found to be a critical contributing factor to brain damage during a stroke. At higher temperatures, the chemical reactions are faster, and the resulting damage is greater. By lowering brain temperature during stroke, doctors may be able to slow down the ischemic process considerably and protect brain tissue that is at risk. But this has not yet been proven to be clinically beneficial.

The acid content of brain cells is also disturbed by ischemia. This results in enzyme malfunctions within the cell that may affect blood flow into the brain. In turn, that problem may prompt edema, or swelling. Some stroke researchers are investigating how to restore the correct acid balance to the cells in time to prevent or reduce cellular death.

Experimental drugs to block the chemical cascade are being developed. One of these is called a **calcium channel blocker.**

Research in this area has proceeded on the theory that permanent brain damage due to stroke may not be caused directly by too little blood or by hemorrhage into the brain. Rather, stroke may damage the brain because either scenario fatally disrupts the delicate chemical balance of brain cells. Such a dramatic imbalance initiates a cascade of chemical reactions in the cell that are the real culprits behind permanent brain damage. An excessive amount of calcium in the brain cells is thought to be one such toxic trigger.

The theory is that if doctors could learn to "block" this cascade before it starts, they could buy time for the cell—time in which to restore normal blood flow and prevent permanent damage. Calcium channel blockers are a type of drug that may protect brain cells from this cascade effect. They may prove beneficial both for hemorrhagic and ischemic stroke patients. Calcium channel blocker drugs have already been proven beneficial to some heart disease patients. But they are still in the experimental stage where stroke is concerned, and they are available only to patients in experimental studies.

Common Complications of Stroke

Stroke is a major illness. It is common to find it complicated by other medical problems. Complications may range from limb contractures, pneumonia, and other physical ailments to depression. In addition, some problems that develop after a stroke may, strictly speaking, have nothing to do with the stroke at all, but they nevertheless require treatment.

The following sections briefly describe some of the more common complications that may follow a stroke. Wherever possible, the best course of action is preventing these complications, rather than treating them after they appear.

Edema

Sometimes after a large stroke due to hemorrhage or infarction, the brain starts to swell, causing a condition known as **brain edema** (pronounced "eh-DEE-ma"). It usually occurs within the first seventy-two hours of the stroke if it happens at all. Brain edema displaces important structures and may cause further brain damage, causing serious new problems for the patient.

Heart Problems

Heart problems and stroke very often go hand in hand, whether the stroke is ischemic or hemorrhagic. Cardiac troubles can cause stroke, especially embolic strokes and TIAs. But heart problems are also commonly found to coexist with stroke conditions and even to be caused by them. It should be no surprise that this is so. The body's cardiovascular system assures that the heart and blood vessels are interdependent in their job of supplying the body with nutrients and oxygen. What affects one element of the system is very likely to affect the other in some way as well.

Small blood clots generated from a dysfunctional heart can be a very serious problem. These emboli, which may have traveled to the brain and caused ischemic stroke, or TIAs, can also travel to other parts of the body. All patients with heart disease are at some risk of this complication, but those most at risk have secondary risk factors that complicate their health profile, such as obesity or congestive heart failure. People recovering from stroke should work with their doctors to develop a program to reduce their risk factors for heart disease as well as for stroke.

Chest pain or **angina** may also be aggravated or caused by the person's extra exertions during rehabilitative therapy and should be treated accordingly.

Blood Vessel Problems

A person who is paralyzed and immobile because of her stroke is also at high risk of blood clots forming in the veins in the affected leg (vein thrombosis). If these clots break away, they can cause a pulmonary embolism. To help prevent this, physicians usually start patients on physical therapy as soon as possible. The patient should be helped to bend and flex the afflicted limbs, and rotate the ankle throughout the day. (Physical therapy is discussed more fully in Chapter Five.) Support hose or special stockings can help maintain proper circulation in the legs. In addition, the physician may put the patient on anticoagulant therapy to discourage the formation of blood clots. This is done only if the patient didn't have a hemor-rhagic stroke or isn't otherwise a poor candidate for that treatment.

Bed Sores

Also called "pressure ulcers," bed sores can develop if bedridden patients are left too long in one position. Bed sores are completely avoidable with a little preventive attention. Patients should be turned frequently, and they should eat nutritious diets. Their skin should be kept clean and dry. A special mattress or padding in the bed may help, too. If sores do develop, all pressure on them must be eliminated and they should be covered with a sterile dressing.

Limb Contractures

Arms and legs on the paralyzed side of some stroke survivors have a tendency to cramp and "freeze" in position over time if they are not taken through range-of-motion exercises regularly and kept limber. A **painful shoulder** can result from a weak or paralyzed arm that isn't properly supported. Sometimes an inflammation of the shoulder joint occurs. The result is a very painful condition called **"frozen" shoulder.** Fortunately, limb contractures can be easily avoided if physical therapy is started right from the patient's bedside soon after a stroke. Physical therapy is discussed in greater depth in the next chapter.

Arthritis

Arthritis may develop in the joints on the side of the body affected by the stroke. Immobility of those limbs can cause muscle loss around those joints. Physical therapy and aspirin therapy, super-vised by the doctor, help manage this condition.

Pneumonia

Pneumonia is a common complication of many major illnesses, including stroke. It generally develops within one to three weeks of the stroke. People who have difficulty breathing or swallowing properly as a result of their strokes are at special risk. Deep breathing exercises and frequent coughing help prevent pneumonia. Walking as soon as possible, or being turned frequently if bedridden, also helps.

Seizures

About 10 percent of those who have a stroke later have seizures. Fortunately, this complication isn't permanent for most people. Most of these episodes occur in the first day or two after stroke. They are attributed to brain scars left after the stroke. Such seizures usually can be controlled with anticonvulsant medication.

Urinary Tract Infection and Bladder Control

The urinary tract is a common site for infection after stroke. There can be many reasons for the problem's developing. Occasionally a person's ability to control his bladder is affected by a stroke. This can cause infections, but the condition is usually temporary, unless the stroke was very large. A person who has had a stroke should be encouraged to visit the bathroom frequently, day and night, to retrain the bladder.

Sometimes the real problem is not a matter of bladder control at all, but of communication. Some stroke survivors may languish because they cannot get to the bathroom without physical help and cannot ask for it. People with aphasia may have difficulty because they can't clearly communicate their needs to others. Just a little extra thought and attention from caregivers and family members to these possible problems can go a long way toward solving them. In Chapters Six and Seven we will give you some ideas for helping those who are physically disabled and for communicating with people with aphasia.

Depression

Depression is a common by-product of stroke and is estimated to affect up to two-fifths of all stroke survivors. However, sometimes this condition has a physical rather than an emotional source.

Some stroke outcomes mimic the signs of depression. For example, a person who is unable because of a brain injury to inject emotion into his voice sounds depressed as a result. Others can't control laughing or crying after a stroke. They may cry uncontrollably until they are interrupted—and then they may stop abruptly and return to normal again. These people may not be depressed in the true sense, either.

But, certainly, having a new disability or change in circumstance brought about by stroke can trigger an emotional depression. Stroke survivors may feel unhappy about their condition and helpless in their disabilities. They may grieve over their loss of competence. Pride and self-image may also be damaged. Many stroke survivors feel a loss of power and control over their lives. They may be pessimistic about the future.

Depression can interfere with a person's progress in rehabilitation, and it can create behavioral problems.

Typical signs of depression include:

> Personality change
> Emotional outbursts
> Irritability
> Rudeness
> Suicidal thoughts
> Wide variations in appetite
> Wide variations in sleep
> Unwillingness to communicate
> Inability to enjoy life
> Slower-than-expected recovery
> Lack of cooperation in rehabilitation

Some stroke survivors talk about feeling depressed, but others withdraw into silence. Depression can cause a continual sense of emotional pain and deprive people of their happiness.

There is hope, however. Most stroke survivors who experience depression recover fully and regain their joy of life. They accept their condition and their disabilities. They find satisfaction in achieving new goals and compensating for abilities they have lost.

Family and caregivers can help someone recovering from stroke by maintaining an upbeat attitude. They can help him regain self-confidence by emphasizing the ways in which he can restore his independence through rehabilitation therapy. Plenty of affection, attention, understanding, and respect help, too. Individual therapy or support groups can help in many cases—especially when the stroke survivor feels isolated or pessimistic. Some people who have not responded to other forms of treatment may need antidepressant medication. Short-term treatment with these medications is usually very successful for these people.

Depression can be a problem for caregivers, too. Their lives also have been disrupted by their loved one's stroke. Counseling or a support group may be helpful. Depression is discussed in greater detail in Chapter Seven.

Ike had been a farmer all his life, when, at sixty-five, he had a major stroke that left him with partial paralysis on the right side of his body. Suddenly Ike couldn't do the things he had always done. He felt stripped of the independence he had always been so fiercely proud of. Despite the encouragement of his wife and family, Ike withdrew into himself. He refused to go to physical therapy at the hospital or even to try to get out of bed.

Ike's family saw how depressed he was becoming, but nothing they could say seemed to change his hopeless view of his situation. He didn't even show any interest in news of the farm. Sometimes he even snapped at them, which was wholly out of character for this usually gentle man.

One morning, on a routine visit, Ike's wife, Ruth, found Ike in extreme pain. "It's my shoulder," he said gruffly. "It hurts like heck and I can't move the darn thing at all."

Nurses on the floor had already noticed this development and had called in Ike's attending physician. She immediately arranged for intensive therapy to get Ike's shoulder moving again. Despite the pain he felt, however, Ike still stubbornly refused to participate.

Dr. Curtis sat down with her patient and talked with him for a long time. Later, she spoke with Ruth.

"Ike is a proud man, and this stroke has obviously hit him hard. I think physical and occupational therapy can really help him. He can learn some new skills to compensate for his deficits. Then I think he'll bounce back. But for a little while, I'd like to treat him with some antidepressant medication. Don't worry, it's not unusual for a person who has had a stroke to feel depressed afterward. It usually goes away. The medication, though, will help us get him into the therapy he must have immediately to restore mobility to his shoulder. And it should get him into a more hopeful frame of mind about a lot of things. Your husband is very lucky to be alive. I know that once he's feeling a little better, he'll realize it.

"You and your children can help," Dr. Curtis continued. "I'd like to sign you all up to learn some of the range-of-mobility exercises we need Ike to practice every day. Then you and your kids can participate in this activity with him. You'll all feel happier, I think, if you can help him a little with this. The first thing we need to do is get his frozen shoulder taken care of. Ike's potential for recovery is really very good. We just have to help him see that!"

The Next Step

After the immediate crisis of the stroke has passed and the stroke survivor has stabilized medically, a new phase begins. It is time for the physician, stroke survivor, and family to consider rehabilitation therapy. That is the subject of our next chapter.

5
Rehabilitation Therapy

For most stroke survivors, rehabilitation therapy is a very important part of their recovery. It restores self-esteem, and it can mean the difference between independence and confinement. Rehabilitation requires a great deal of commitment from everyone involved. This includes the stroke survivor, caregiver, and health care staff. But the rewards are tangible and important.

The aim of any rehabilitation program is to help the survivor adapt to his deficit and to recover as much of his previous independence as possible. Rehabilitation strategies include physical, occupational, and speech therapies. Any or all of these may be used as appropriate.

Rehabilitation helps the great majority of stroke survivors avoid nursing home care and return home. Almost a third of all stroke survivors who work return to their jobs within a year of their strokes. It is estimated that by the end of that first year, more than half of all stroke survivors need no assistance at all in their daily living tasks. Just 20 percent continue to need help for complex tasks only, such as bathing. While about 15 percent become more dependent on others than they were before their strokes, only 5 percent become completely dependent on others. Some survivors even do some of their best work after their strokes. One example is Louis Pasteur, the French chemist who pioneered the field of bacteriology. President Dwight D. Eisenhower is another famous man who enjoyed continued success after his stroke. There is no doubt that recovery after stroke can be substantial.

Rehabilitation therapy can be an important factor to that recovery. The intensity of therapy varies, depending on the stroke survivor's degree of disability. Even the best rehabilitation program, however, won't return people to *exactly* what they were before the stroke. In most cases, that just isn't a reasonable expectation, and to anticipate it only results in frustration. In fact, in most cases, recovering exactly the same skills one had before isn't necessary. New ways to complete old tasks can be learned through rehabilitation therapy.

The goal of rehabilitation therapy is to help people adapt to their deficits, not get rid of them. Rehabilitation therapy does not change the neurological deficit that occurred at the time of the stroke. That isn't possible. Most people do spontaneously recover some lost brain function within a few hours or months after their strokes, depending on the strokes' severity. After that relatively short period, however, some deficit usually persists. It can be overcome with the help of rehabilitation therapy in many cases, but it cannot be cured or otherwise "fixed."

The Rehabilitation Team

Most people who have had a stroke require rehabilitation in a number of areas. Several different specialists often combine their skills to provide the most complete recovery program possible. (A typical rehabilitation team is described on page 140.) For best results, a rehab program should be coordinated among the specialists involved. It should also be fully integrated with the medical care the person receives.

Usually, the physician in charge of the patient's case at the hospital heads the team, answering any questions and resolving any conflicts. But others, usually the family and a rehabilitation nurse assigned to the case, take care of the day-to-day coordination of the stroke survivor's activities.

The rehabilitation team should be assembled as soon as possible after the patient has stabilized, and it should meet regularly thereafter. Regular meetings give all members the chance to form joint goals and coordinate their strategies. It also gives each person an

---

THE REHABILITATION THERAPY TEAM

A typical rehabilitation program for a person who has had a stroke may involve a number of professionals. Each one works with the stroke survivor on different areas of recovery. Studies have shown that the person's overall progress is enhanced if these specialists coordinate their efforts on his behalf.

The list below includes many people who might be considered part of the rehabilitation team. Not every person in rehabilitation may need all the services implied by this list. The physician in charge will suggest a team best suited to the individual's needs.

> Stroke survivor
> Stroke survivor's family
> Primary or attending physician to the stroke survivor
> Medical specialists
> Dietitian/Nutritionist
> Rehabilitation nurse
> Physical therapist
> Occupational therapist
> Vocational therapist
> Speech specialist
> Recreational therapist
> Social worker
> Psychologists

---

opportunity to compare notes with other professionals and to share information about and insights into the individual case. These meetings should continue as long as necessary. They may still be useful after the stroke survivor is moved from acute care to the rehabilitation ward of the hospital, for example, or from the hospital to home.

Formal organization of such stroke teams does improve the stroke survivor's ultimate recovery outcome. The family of the person in a rehab program should discuss the team with the attending physician or rehabilitation nurse.

The Family's Role

A stroke always affects more than one person. Often the families or close friends of stroke survivors find their lives turned upside down, too, as they adjust to their loved one's post-stroke condition. New roles may be forged among family members very suddenly, with new responsibilities. Not all of these roles are welcome, and some take getting used to. A stressful environment for stroke survivor *and* family can result.

But direct participation in the person's rehab program can diffuse some tensions and make transitions easier for everyone. Working toward a common goal can promote communication and reduce conflict among family members. Many important rehabilitation techniques can be carried out at home. Family involvement also reemphasizes to the stroke survivor, whose self-esteem may be low, that he is still very important to his loved ones.

The family and friends of the stroke survivor can contribute to the rehabilitative process in two particularly significant ways. They can help with rehabilitation exercises and in the active coordination of the day-to-day program. Equally important, they can provide strong emotional support throughout the rehabilitation program. They can encourage the stroke survivor often and remind him of how much he is needed by family and friends.

A therapist can spend only a limited amount of time with the stroke survivor each week. Trained family members, however, can continue to work throughout the day with their loved one who has had a stroke. This can be done without the therapist present, at the hospital and at home. Caregivers can ask the therapists who will be working with the stroke survivor and designing his program what they can do to help.

It is a particularly good idea for a caregiver to learn the ropes while the patient is still at the hospital and professionals are nearby. Therapists and rehabilitative nurses are available there both to answer questions and to monitor results. One family member might even find it useful to stay at the hospital with the patient for a few days before discharge. At the hospital, the caregiver can get acquainted with the patient's new routines and help with rehabilitation exercises under the therapist's supervision.

Perhaps the most important contribution every family member

can make, however, is to maintain an upbeat, optimistic attitude around the stroke survivor. That isn't always easy; caregivers have hard days, too. But being cheerful makes a positive difference.

When working with a loved one who has had a stroke, it's perfectly all right to show empathy for a person who is having difficulty with some of the exercises. But also help him focus on the benefits of mastering the various exercises. Keep goals practical and within his reach. Praise success often, but don't praise without reason. Doing so only makes you look patronizing, and your loved one will feel let down—or, worse, confused. Keep your own spirits up, and recognize the importance of your role in the stroke patient's rehabilitation.

Stroke survivors and caregivers may benefit from getting together with others with similar experiences. A stroke club offers an opportunity to do that. For information on stroke clubs, contact the American Heart Association's Stroke Connection (see page 290).

Diane had had a major stroke a month before, but she seemed to be making a strong recovery, which was a great relief to her husband and grown children. She did still have persistent weakness on her left side, however.

In the weeks following the stroke, Dr. Estavez, Diane, her husband, Keith, and other members of their family had regular discussions about Diane and her progress. In one of these discussions, five weeks after the stroke, Dr. Estavez suggested that it was time to think about getting Diane into a rehabilitation program. He said that proper rehabilitation would teach her to compensate for her remaining deficits and restore her to the maximum independence possible.

"I'm sure Diane will benefit from rehabilitation therapy," Dr. Estavez told the family. "I'd like to set up a rehab team for her, of which I'll be the head. As you've learned, stroke is a complicated illness. It affects a number of functions, which can overlap. That's why a team of experts, working together, can be so effective for a stroke survivor's maximum rehabilitation outlook. Each member of the team is an expert in a different area. I'd like you to meet them all. I think for Diane, we'll have occupational, physical, vocational, and speech specialists, a registered dietitian, her rehabilitation nurse, and a psychologist working with her. We'll also have the medical specialists she's already seeing.

"What we'll do is meet on a regular basis to discuss Diane's case with each other. A rehab team shares information about the stroke survivor as the rehabilitation is in progress. Then we coordinate our activities for maximum effectiveness on behalf of the stroke survivor. We've found it to be a very successful way to handle a person's rehab program.

"I'd like to put you and your children on the team, too, Keith," Dr. Estavez continued. "The family may be the most important part of this team. Diane will need your encouragement at every step, because some of what she will be learning will take time. It won't be easy or fast. She's likely to become frustrated sometimes. Can I count on you?"

"Diane's always been a team player, and so are we," said Keith, speaking for the whole family. "Let's get started!"

Factors That May Influence Success

Even with the best rehabilitation team and most supportive family, the success of a rehabilitation program can depend on a number of factors. First among them are the cause, size, and location of the stroke. Beyond that, success depends on the therapy itself and also on the health and responsiveness of the stroke survivor.

The Therapy Itself

In general, the most successful therapy does the following:

- Begins very soon after the stroke, even at the patient's bedside. Range-of-motion exercises are done simply to keep tendons and ligaments flexible and toned until more active physical therapy can begin.
- Starts with simple exercises and builds logically to more complicated tasks.
- Addresses the stroke survivor's needs. These needs

may include physical, occupational, speech, and even psychological therapy. These are viewed as parts of one larger, coordinated treatment plan. The different therapists and doctors involved in the patient's care are kept informed of each other's progress. Usually the person's original physician heads this "stroke team."

- Is carefully tailored to specific needs of the individual.

The Stroke Survivor's Condition

The most successful therapy also depends on the nature of the person's deficits and her general physical and emotional health. These factors are far more important than the person's age alone, especially in the case of physical therapy. Despite popular perceptions, not every person who has had a stroke needs or benefits from rehabilitation therapy. Those with slight or temporary deficits often can get adequate help from outpatient services at the hospital, if necessary. At the other end of the scale are people who are completely immobilized or otherwise incapacitated by their strokes. These individuals don't usually benefit from rehabilitation therapy. Those who benefit most fall between these two groups.

Stroke survivors who do well in rehab therapy often have the following in common:

- Spontaneous recovery of some voluntary movement soon after the stroke. Physical therapy can build on this movement. The greater the extent of paralysis, the harder it is to regain meaningful movement of the limb.
- No major medical illness, such as heart disease or severe arthritis, in addition to stroke.
- A sense of touch in their paralyzed extremities.
- No sensory or visual impairments (see box on page 146).
- No mental disorders, such as Alzheimer's disease, so they can learn new ways to accomplish daily tasks.
- An ability to understand what is asked of them. People with language problems, such as Wernicke's aphasia, have a more difficult time in rehab therapy.

- Lack of depression, or, if the patients are depressed, a response to treatment.
- A caring, supportive family that is able to participate in rehabilitation therapy with them. This is especially valuable to rehabilitation.

Serious problems in any of these areas can interfere with successful rehabilitation. Rehab programs often require many months of concentrated effort before they reap results. Not every stroke survivor has the stamina for that kind of program.

Each person who has had a stroke is unique, however. Individual factors count, and doctors weigh all pros and cons carefully before recommending a rehabilitation program to the stroke survivor and her family. If there is some question as to whether or not the person may benefit from a rehab program, she will usually be given the opportunity to try it and see. Results of these programs should be monitored carefully. Rehab programs should not be continued when no further results can be expected.

Hazel had a major stroke that left her paralyzed on one side of her body. In the weeks following her stroke, doctors looked for signs of some spontaneous recovery of the functions that she had lost. Unfortunately, there was very little spontaneous recovery observed in her. In addition, Hazel had severe arthritis, which her doctors knew would make physical rehabilitation even more difficult.

Hazel's family was eager for her to try rehabilitation therapy anyway. Arrangements were made for her to begin work with physical therapy specialists at the hospital.

Despite their efforts, however, Hazel's doctor, Dr. Alhambra, observed virtually no improvement in Hazel's voluntary movements over several weeks. It was disappointing, because everyone, from Hazel to her therapists to her family, had worked very hard. When it was clear that further efforts would go nowhere, Dr. Alhambra had a meeting with Hazel and her family to discuss what to do next.

"Rehabilitation therapy just isn't meant for every stroke survivor," Dr. Alhambra told them. "In Hazel's case, she recovered very little voluntary movement spontaneously right after her stroke. This was a sign that we might not be able to expect much recovery—no matter how much rehabilitation therapy we tried. And her arthritis was another factor that suggested her mobility would be hard to recover under any circumstances. But, because sometimes we can be pleasantly surprised, we did think it would be worth trying, just in case. I'm sorry to say that our hopes weren't fulfilled. Continuing would only be tiring and frustrating for Hazel at this point, and not a good use of resources, either. I think we've got to reconsider and look in another direction that will yield better results for our efforts.

"Hazel will stop going to physical therapy to recover movement on her right side. However, I do want her to continue going to occupational therapy to learn ways to compensate for those deficits." He turned to Hazel, who was looking disappointed. "There is still much we can do to maximize your self-sufficiency, Hazel. We're just taking your rehabilitation in a slightly different direction."

SENSORY AND VISUAL IMPAIRMENTS

Special problems occur when a person who has had a stroke has deficits such as sensory and visual neglect, in which he ignores one side of his body or one half of his visual field. These can severely disrupt a rehab program, for the simple reason that it is difficult to persuade someone to work on a problem he doesn't recognize. Sensory deficits usually aren't improved by rehabilitation, although they may improve spontaneously. Visual neglect is somewhat more responsive to therapy if it is not accompanied by other sensory deficits. A person with this difficulty can learn to compensate to some degree for it. The deficit itself does not go away, however. Such a person should be restricted from some activities, such as driving, for his own safety as well as that of others.

The Rehabilitation Timeline

Doctors agree that rehabilitation therapy should start as soon as possible after a stroke for best results. No one can say exactly how long a rehabilitation program should last once begun. Each program is designed to meet the specific needs of the individual. Some general guidelines do exist, however.

Immediate Measures

In the first two to three days, up to the first few weeks, the main goal of rehabilitation is to prevent the person's joints and muscles in any paralyzed limbs from contracting. Visual and sensory deficits are dealt with later. In the three weeks following a stroke, recovery of all kinds varies widely. Some patients may note a good deal of improvement in movement, aphasia (difficulty with speech and language), vision, sensory perception, and other areas. Others may show slower progress in that time.

Patients are encouraged to get out of bed a day or two after their strokes if they can do so safely. Those with other serious medical problems, including diabetes or heart disease, might be kept in bed four or five days. (Patients who have not recovered full consciousness are another logical exception to this rule.) Lengthy bed rest is discouraged for the majority of patients because it can invite other problems, including pneumonia or heart attack resulting from emboli from veins in the legs. At the least, most people should sit up in a chair within a couple of days of their strokes. Sitting up is good for emotional outlook as well as health.

Intermediate Measures

After a few weeks, the progress of the stroke survivor's recovery becomes more standardized. During this phase, the degree of the person's disability is assessed. Muscle tone is tested at regular intervals. Motor functions, which include activities of daily living (ADLs), are checked out. ADLs are basic self-care tasks. They include the ability to eat, to bathe and dress oneself, to move from bed to chair, to walk and handle steps, to maintain bladder and bowel control and use the toilet, and to speak and understand speech. (These are discussed more fully in Chapter Seven.)

Cognitive functions are also assessed now. These include the ability to learn new ways to remain independent. The size and location of the stroke have a lot to do with cognitive problems. Mood is also carefully monitored, because depression can interfere with the success of a rehab program.

The three to six months following the stroke are considered the most important period for rehabilitative progress. Most significant voluntary movement is usually recovered in the first six months. Speech, steadiness, and daily activity skills may continue to improve significantly for up to two years or even longer after a stroke.

Physical Therapy

The primary goal of physical therapy is to retrain the stroke survivor to walk. This form of rehabilitation therapy starts right at the patient's bedside. A professional in this field is known as a **physical therapist.**

The Prognosis

The physical therapist first evaluates the patient's level of physical disability and the degree of recovery that is likely. The site and size of the brain lesion left by the stroke is the most important factor in this evaluation. Magnetic resonance imaging tests (MRIs), as well as computed tomography (CT scans), can be very helpful in making this diagnosis. Large lesions falling directly on the main motor strip area of the brain give the poorest outlook for motor function recovery. If the lesion falls outside this main area, however, rapid, impressive improvement can sometimes be achieved. (The motor cortex area of the brain is discussed in Chapter One.) Most experts agree that if some function hasn't returned to the afflicted limbs within three weeks of the stroke, there will probably always be some degree of paralysis.

The recovery outlook also changes if other deficits are involved. A stroke survivor who has only a motor deficit is likely to become independently ambulatory within fourteen weeks of his stroke. If for some other reason he hasn't made significant progress toward that goal within that time, however, the odds are not good that he will ever walk independently again.

If he has sensory deficits, too (such as neglect), his chances of walking independently again start to get worse, down to about one in three. Finally, if he has combined motor, sensory, and visual deficits after his stroke, he probably cannot expect to walk independently again. He may, however, eventually learn to walk with some support devices.

After evaluation, a strategy is devised for the stroke survivor. It has three goals: to help the individual regain some function, to maintain remaining function, and to teach compensatory functions. The physical therapist considers the person's unimpaired side when developing a rehab program. Those limbs often can be trained to take over some of the tasks formerly done by the impaired side.

Immediate Measures

The physical therapist's immediate concern for stroke survivors is to keep any weakened or paralyzed limbs flexible. This serves two purposes. First, it prevents muscles and joints in the afflicted limbs from stiffening and contracting through disuse. This kind of problem is often called a **contracture.** This painful complication can make rehabilitation of the limbs much harder later on. Second, the activity begins the process of stimulating and developing areas in the brain that were previously unused for this purpose to take over and compensate for some lost functions. The brain seems to respond to this kind of "rewiring" best if the exercises are repeated frequently and are initiated as soon as possible after the stroke.

To keep joints flexible, physical therapists start patients on a program of **range-of-motion exercises.** Pain and stiffness can begin to develop in the first few hours after the stroke, so this element of the recovery program starts almost immediately. Range-of-motion exercises are passive, meaning that the limb itself doesn't exert effort (to lift itself, for example). The physical therapist moves the patient's affected limbs, fingers, and toes through a full range of gentle bending movements. At rest, the patient's fingers are usually arranged around a rolled towel so that they don't cramp up and become fixed in that position.

All joints on the paralyzed side of the body should be taken through this routine three or four times daily, depending on the physical therapist's recommendations. Nurses and family members can learn the routine easily and be of enormous help in making sure the patient gets enough of these "workouts." Sometimes even the patient himself may use his well arm to move the impaired limbs through the exercises.

Range-of-motion exercises also help the stroke survivor prepare for the more demanding physical and occupational therapies to follow. They have nothing to do with helping the person regain specific skills, however. That comes later.

Sometimes, despite an early program of range-of-motion exercises, spasticity develops in the affected limbs. **Spasticity** is the increased resistance to passive motion of the involved arms and legs. A spastic limb is difficult to move, and it may hurt when it is moved. Spasticity can be a serious problem for the stroke survivor. Besides being painful, it makes it difficult for him to go on to other important physical therapy exercises.

Unfortunately, there isn't a surefire way to prevent spasticity from developing, but range-of-motion exercises do help. Once spasticity is detected, however, doctors can rely on a number of targeted therapies to relieve the condition. These range from muscle relaxants and heat therapies to massage and acupuncture.

Painful and "frozen" shoulder are two related complications of paralysis. Fortunately, they are easily prevented. Painful shoulder is caused by the unsupported weight of a weak or paralyzed arm stretching and pulling the muscles of the shoulder. This stretching also affects the shoulder joint capsule. It eventually pulls the arm joint from the shoulder socket altogether and causes a dislocation. To avoid these problems, the paralyzed arm is usually supported when the stroke survivor sits up. To encourage circulation, the arm is kept at the level of or slightly higher than the heart.

Frozen shoulder is a related condition, identified by inflammation of the shoulder joint, which develops within several hours of the stroke. A frozen shoulder causes constant pain and severe stiffness. The pain becomes worse if the arm is moved. Frequent range-of-motion exercises help prevent frozen shoulder. If frozen shoulder does develop, however, the condition can be treated with medication.

Circulation is affected, especially in the legs, by long periods of immobility. Blood clots may form in the veins of the legs. If these clots break away and are carried back to the heart, they can cause a pulmonary embolism. Range-of-motion exercises help prevent this by stimulating circulation. Raising the patient's legs slightly in bed can also help prevent this complication. If he is sitting, raising his legs to the level of the chair seat can help. A paralyzed arm may be fixed in a sling that holds it at the level of the heart or higher.

A stroke involving the brain stem might cause a person to have double vision or an eyelid droop. Double vision is generally treated with an eye patch. A droopy eyelid may be propped up by special devices, but normal blinking can't be restored.

Intermediate and Long-Term Measures

When the stroke survivor has recovered some strength and movement, it is literally time for the next step. The physical therapist will now concentrate on helping the person walk again. Most people whose strokes caused paralysis in the upper part of the body tend to retain some movement in their legs. They usually can learn to walk, alone or with the help of support devices. The therapist will look at the degree of strength and voluntary movement that remains in the person's lower extremities. This determines to a large extent whether the person is likely to walk completely independently or not. But even if the return of voluntary movement is slight, the stroke survivor may still be able to walk with the use of braces, canes, or other supportive devices. Walking, with or without support, is always a desirable goal for the patient, for it represents personal independence.

The physical therapist must prepare the stroke survivor for standing, walking, or transferring from bed to wheelchair. A number of exercises may be used. Some focus on balance and shifting body weight, and others strengthen muscles and build endurance.

A familiar adage says we all must learn how to walk before we can run. Physical therapists would agree, but might add that a person who has had a stroke must also learn how to stand before he can walk. Once the stroke survivor is able to stand, his therapist can determine his stability on the impaired side. He can also be fitted with an appropriate brace if needed.

Next, the physical therapist checks for any weakness in the impaired leg, which commonly causes the foot to turn inward as unused muscles contract. This condition, called **foot drop,** can be corrected with a foot brace. The brace picks up the toes so that the person is able to take a step. Corrective shoes may also provide greater stability in conjunction with the brace.

The stroke survivor usually starts walking in the hospital. At first he may use special equipment called parallel bars. These waist-high bars form a narrow aisle across part of a room. The stroke survivor uses the bars to help support himself as he practices walking between them.

After he builds up strength in his legs, the stroke survivor typically graduates to walking outside of parallel bars, leaning on a therapist or two instead for arm support. After he masters that, he can be fitted with a cane or walker—and he's on his way to renewed independence.

Doris had had a major stroke. A physical therapist began range-of-motion exercises with her as soon as she was stabilized. Doris continued these exercises several times a day while bedridden. The physical therapist taught Doris's grown children how to help with the exercises. They took turns with the physical therapist in doing these exercises with Doris.

In the weeks following her stroke, Doris continued to improve. Consequently, her physical therapy exercises became more intensive. She learned to sit up and then to move from her bed to a chair. With an occupational therapist, she learned to eat with her left hand instead of her right, which was compromised by the stroke. She worked with her therapists on becoming stronger.

Her physical therapy specialist was very pleased with her progress. "Doris, I think it's time for us to kick you out of the hospital and send you home! Do you live alone or with anyone?"

"I do live alone," Doris said, "but my daughter would stay with me for a while. We talked about it. If it looks like I can handle it after a few weeks, we thought maybe we could just check in with each other by phone every day at some regular time after that. She lives here in town. Is that OK?"

"We'll have to talk with the rest of your rehab team, of course, but that sounds fine to me. Your progress has been really good. Some of us would like to visit your house before you go home, though. This is so we can make safety and adaptation recommendations for it that can be carried out before you get there. We need to be sure that at least some of the house is wheelchair-accessible for you. Shall I schedule that visit for early next week?"

Doris beamed. "Or sooner," she suggested pointedly.

Back at home, Doris found everything the same and yet very different. Although her rehabilitation team had done a good job in adapting much of the house to her particular deficits, some activities continued to frustrate her. Making dinner with one hand was a slow process, even with adaptive equipment. But she was glad to be home, watering her own plants and surrounded by her own things. And she was eager to try walking as soon as possible. Practicing with a visiting therapist and her daughter as her strength allowed took up much of Doris's time.

Three and a half months after her stroke, Doris is ready to stand and walk again, using a three-footed walker. It is hard work for this older woman, and there are days when everything seems to go wrong. But she perseveres. Her walking is becoming more confident. She summed it up for her daughter during one of their regular calls.

"You know, my life isn't the same as it was before the stroke, but it certainly isn't bad, either. It's even kind of a challenge to find new ways to do some of the same old jobs around this house. They had gotten to be so boring!"

Palsies

Strokes along the motor strip in the brain's cerebrum and its related structures can result in the kinds of weakness and paralysis that are discussed above. Many of our involuntary movements originate in the brain stem. Strokes there can also disturb a person's ability to walk. With some brain stem strokes, the person still retains the strength and ability to walk. But her gait, or the way she walks, is disturbed.

This problem mainly manifests itself in two ways. **Disequilibrium** can afflict those with brain stem lesions. In this case, the person has a difficult time maintaining her balance as she walks. Her steps are uncertain and she may fall often. Although this problem doesn't go away, usually the person learns to compensate for it within a month or two. Her walking will not be permanently affected. **Ataxia** is a less common but more serious problem. Ataxia is a condition in which muscle coordination fails or becomes extremely irregular. Unfortunately, physical therapy does not help people who have this condition. They can often walk but are clumsy and may need some form of support.

Occupational Therapy

Physical therapy might be defined as rehabilitation therapy that addresses the lower body. **Occupational therapy** (OT), on the other hand, could be defined as therapy that addresses the upper body. Any rehab program should include occupational therapy.

OT is concerned with helping the stroke survivor readapt to everyday life. The aim here is to rehabilitate the practical skills needed at home and at one's job and to restore the person's independence as far as possible. A specialist in this field is called an **occupational therapist.**

After Yuan had a thrombotic stroke, the left side of his body remained weak. A fifty-year-old dentist, Yuan was determined that this setback would not keep him from returning to his beloved practice.

With the help of an occupational therapy specialist, Yuan worked to strengthen his left side and recover some of the voluntary movements he had lost, especially in his hand. After some weeks of intensive therapy, Yuan showed a great deal of improvement. Despite this, some weakness remained in his hand. One day, his partner in the dental practice stopped by Yuan's house for lunch. He found Yuan in a subdued mood.

"I've made a lot of improvement, Randy, but they're telling me I've probably gone as far as therapy can take me. I still don't have the fine motor coordination in my hand that I used to. How can I perform surgery now? I don't know if I should retire early or what. I certainly don't want to!"

Randy leaned back in his chair and eyed his old friend and business partner. "Yuan, you should know me better than that. I wouldn't let you retire. I know you don't want to. You had talked about easing up on your work schedule a bit, even before your stroke. Let's just slow down and think about how we might adapt to each other a bit here."

In the weeks that followed, the two men did talk. Eventually they decided that Randy would take over all surgeries and fillings. They decided Yuan would evaluate all X rays, perform examinations, and consult with the patients.

"I am glad to be able to focus on the technical aspects of dentistry, Yuan. You were always better at explaining procedures to our patients, anyway," Randy said.

"I think I'll like my new role," Yuan said.

"This new division of duties is going to work out just fine— for us and our patients," Randy reassured him.

Prognosis

How much progress can be expected from occupational therapy depends on how much strength the person has retained in his upper body after the stroke. The weaker his motor coordination, the less likely it is that he will be able to recover fully. And if the dominant hand has been affected by the stroke, the person may permanently lose the ability to perform some activities with that hand, such as writing or buttoning a shirt. Fortunately, most of these activities can be learned and accomplished by the unimpaired hand with the help of occupational therapy.

Immediate Goals

Not surprisingly, the first thing a stroke survivor with a weak or paralyzed arm needs to learn after a stroke is how to sit up in bed safely. That task is followed closely by how to get out of bed safely. Initially, a trapeze bar or a soft rope tied to the end of the bed or suspended above the person is helpful. The person can simply reach for it with his unimpaired arm and pull himself upright. From there he can pull himself to the side of the bed and swing his legs down. Working with an occupational therapist, he can practice doing this without the bar or rope. Practice helps him improve his balance and strength. Eventually he will be able to discard supports and sit up without help.

Intermediate and Long-Term Goals

One of the more important tasks the stroke survivor needs to master in this period is called a transfer. *Transfer* is simply a term for the transition a person makes to move from bed to chair, wheelchair to shower, etc. Depending on the degree of the disability, this can be a simple matter or a relatively complicated one that requires learning a new skill.

Transfers can be done standing up if the person has retained enough leg strength after her stroke to permit it. If the legs are impaired, however, transfers can still be made using a sliding board. Sliding boards are positioned between, for example, the bed and a chair. They allow the person to "slide" from one to the other while supported by the board.

An occupational therapist helps prepare a stroke survivor for a sliding transfer. First he prescribes exercises that build up the person's upper arm strength. The therapist at first helps the person practice making transfers. With practice, the stroke survivor's balance improves. She learns to judge the trustworthiness of her weakened limbs in making each transfer and to compensate for them. Eventually she can make transfers alone.

Occupational therapy goes beyond transfers. It also helps people to reacquire skills for a variety of daily activities. Mastery of these skills is important to maintaining independence. Eating, grooming, and cooking are all skills the occupational therapist will address, among others. In many cases, he will introduce the stroke survivor to tools that can make completing the tasks much easier. These include utensil holders and devices that allow one to reach for and grab objects. While the therapist will teach some of these exercises at the hospital, it helps if he can visit the stroke survivor's home and customize techniques as necessary.

The therapist can also give valuable suggestions about how to make adaptations in the home for the stroke survivor's convenience. There are many objects that can make life much easier for those with motor deficits in the hands and arms. Rails along walls, bigger handles on doors and cupboards, tub benches, and hand-held shower heads are just some of them.

Having to relearn skills such as combing one's hair or sipping soup from a spoon—once taken for granted—would be a frustrating, time-consuming experience for anyone. Stroke survivors undergoing occupational therapy need the support and involvement of their loved ones. Caregivers can be taught by the therapist to oversee the stroke survivor's daily practice routine.

Loved ones can also motivate the stroke survivor with encouraging behavior and optimistic words. This is an extremely important role. Many people become discouraged during occupational therapy because the exercises won't make them "just the way they were." It's important to emphasize to them that, even where original function can't be recovered, many alternative ways to compensate for those movements do exist and can be mastered. It's quite possible to learn to accomplish the same goals from a different direction. In the long run, these skills represent important personal independence.

Near the end of summer, not long after his two grandsons had spent a week with him, Hugh had a stroke. It affected a small area in the deep part of the left hemisphere of his brain. His stroke had left him with paralysis on the right side of his body. Since then, he had worked almost every day with therapists. He had retained flexibility in his affected joints and maximized remaining function and strength in those limbs.

A few months after his stroke, Hugh knew he couldn't expect to regain all the movements and functions he had once had. He might not be able to hike in the mountains anymore. But his rehabilitation was still largely successful. Many tasks that he used to do with his right hand he discovered he could do almost as well with his left hand. Other tasks were made easier by using modified equipment suggested by his therapist. Hugh became quite creative in finding new ways to compensate for his remaining weakness on the right side.

Most of all, Hugh was reassured to learn that he could preserve much of his treasured independence, despite his stroke. The therapist at the rehabilitation center had been encouraging and had taught Hugh new skills to use in his daily life. Four months after his stroke, Hugh had learned how to use his strong side and a board to move independently. He could move from his bed to his wheelchair, and from the wheelchair to other places around the house, including the bathroom.

Hugh's success was due in part to the many hours he spent in therapy, the work and encouragement of the therapists, and his determination to be independent. He also had something to look forward to. His grandchildren were coming for another visit. This time they were only spending the weekend. Hugh wouldn't be able to go hiking with them, but the three of them could still be together and enjoy the mountain sunsets from the porch.

Speech Therapy

Aphasia—difficulty with speech and language—commonly appears in stroke survivors with right arm and leg weakness (stroke involving the left cerebral hemisphere). Occasionally speech may be affected by strokes in the brain stem. Speech and language are two related but distinct elements of human communication, and they may not be affected equally by a stroke. Some people who can't speak, for example, can still understand what others say to them. And some who have lost the ability to understand speech may still be able to comprehend what others "say" through their body language.

We put such emphasis on speech as an essential part of human communication that it's easy to consider a person who has lost the ability to speak as more disabled than he really is. In many cases, however, other ways to communicate can be found that work well. Some people with aphasia, for example, can communicate better by writing or reading than by speaking or listening. Others do better with purely visual communication, such as pantomime.

Prognosis

The coordinated efforts of two or three important zones in the dominant cerebral hemisphere (usually the left) make speech and language possible. A severe stroke that affects all three areas results in serious, permanent speech defects. But if the brain lesion is small —that is, if the stroke is mild—a great deal of recovery is often possible.

Sometimes irregularities in speech result from a stroke involving the brain stem, rather than the cerebrum. Signals from all parts of the brain pass through the brain stem on their way out of the skull. A stroke involving this part of the brain can cause "crossed wires" and "mixed signals" to occur. Although such speech defects can be very noticeable at first, they tend to resolve themselves almost completely over time. By then, generally only the stroke survivor himself remains aware of them. No one else notices.

Aphasias can involve both speaking and comprehension difficulties with speech. Rehabilitation is much more difficult for those who can't understand communication, whether spoken, written, or gestured. People with this kind of sensory aphasia can still derive some benefit from a rehabilitation program, and they should be given the opportunity.

Associated problems from the stroke, such as sensory or visual neglect, can also make rehabilitation more difficult. Over time, these problems tend to improve on their own, making speech therapy easier.

There is some disagreement on the extent to which speech therapists are able to *restore* communication function. Most believe that any recovery is spontaneous and can't be restored by learning certain techniques. But speech specialists are still important to rehabilitation for a number of reasons. Their involvement may speed up the natural process of speech recovery, and they can provide strong emotional support. They can be invaluable in helping stroke survivors improve the communication skills that do remain. They can also recommend practical tips that maximize communication between the stroke survivor and others. Speech specialists may also help evaluate and treat other associated problems, such as difficulty swallowing **(dysphagia)**.

Immediate Goals

Language recovery can occur spontaneously during the first three months after the stroke. But rather than take a wait-and-see attitude toward recovery, speech specialists begin soon after the stroke to work with whatever communications skills remain. The particular strategy they employ depends on the person's deficit. Speech specialists may rely on nonverbal, rather than verbal, communication techniques. They may use gestures, body language, facial expressions, or pictures. Or they may use computers and other electronic devices to improve communication with stroke survivors. One device commonly used is called a *word board*. Word boards show single words or short phrases that a person can point to in order to communicate with others. Word boards, of course, work best with those who know what they want to say but have an impairment that prevents them from forming the words themselves. Most speech specialists work out individualized programs for each patient in the first few months following stroke. These programs capitalize on the patient's communications skills. The specialist then shares with the patient's family and medical team some successful strategies for communicating with the patient. Finding some way to communicate with the stroke survivor—even if it is not a traditional way—is extremely important. It helps break down the sense of isolation a person with a speech deficit often feels, and it can help make sure all of the person's needs are met promptly.

Intermediate and Long-Range Goals

Once the three-month period passes and the stroke survivor's speech recovery stabilizes, the role of the speech specialist changes slightly. Now the goal is to maximize the person's remaining language function. Strategies for this vary, depending on the person's deficit. Speech specialists continue to play an important emotional role in this period, too. They can remind a frustrated person to slow down, relax, and enunciate clearly to make her point, and teach her techniques for doing so.

Golda was a woman in her sixties who had had a stroke and was aphasic as a result. In the first two weeks after her stroke,

Golda would try to talk to family members and the hospital staff, but it never came out sensibly. Sometimes she cursed, too, which she had never done before. Frustrated because she wasn't making herself understood, Golda soon stopped trying to communicate altogether.

Her brothers, sisters, nieces, and nephews all came to visit to cheer her up and try to get her to talk. Nothing seemed to work, however, and they were becoming frustrated themselves. They didn't know what to do. They set up a consultation with Golda's doctor.

Dr. Washington called in a speech specialist to evaluate Golda and try to determine a course of therapy for her. Connie began working intensively with Golda. Her goal was to find some method by which Golda might be encouraged to start communicating again, despite her expressive aphasia.

Pantomime and gesturing didn't do it. Neither did pointing at pictures. Neither did singing words instead of speaking them. But Golda did show an interest in word boards. Connie brought in a variety of word boards for Golda to try, some electronic, some not. The word board that worked best for Golda showed short phrases at which she could point to express a thought.

Using the word board has given Golda a new interest in trying to communicate with others. She has begun trying to speak again. With Connie's help, she has learned to stick to simple words and sentences most of the time. She can now communicate with family members who had been so concerned about her in recent weeks. Sometimes, when she gets frustrated, her family reminds her to relax and to speak clearly. She listens to that advice and continues to show improvement.

Going Home

Stroke survivors who have improved and can be taken care of at home are discharged from the hospital. Almost all of them do return home after their rehabilitation programs at the hospital, able to accomplish their daily activities either completely or relatively independently. If a stroke survivor has not improved enough to return to his own home after a period of time, the doctor may recommend a nursing home. But that is a decision to be made by the family with the doctor's help. (Nursing home care is discussed in Chapter Six.)

Some members of the stroke team formed at the hospital may stay in touch with the stroke survivor after he goes home. They may continue to monitor his progress, checking for problems and devising solutions to them, if necessary. Some therapists visit the stroke survivor at home. Others arrange to see him or a family member in their offices. These professionals are valuable resources for the stroke survivor and the family.

Whether a person who has had a stroke will do well back at home can depend on some important supporting factors. Was he able to care for himself before he had his stroke? If not, he probably won't be able to care for himself now. Is there a spouse or other significant person at home? A caring and capable person, one who helps and encourages the stroke survivor to return to his former activities, is crucial. The person who has had a stroke may need special equipment for his home. Can he afford it? If he can drive, does he have a car? If he can't drive, is other transportation available to him so that he can get to the grocery, the pharmacy, the doctor's office, or church?

The home itself may need some modification before the stroke survivor comes home. Can the house be made wheelchair accessible, if necessary? Do stairs pose a problem? Are ramps needed? Is there a bathroom on every floor, and are they wheelchair-accessible? For those who can't get out to the grocery easily, are there stores nearby that will deliver food?

When all the arrangements are made and the stroke survivor is able to leave the hospital, the next phase of treatment and recovery begins. At home he can start to get back into his life. Now is the time to put into practice the skills developed in rehabilitation. It is to that challenge we turn next.

6

After
the Hospital

W hen a stroke survivor is discharged from the hospital, a new chapter opens in his recovery. At the hospital, the patient's medical condition was stabilized, he may have begun rehabilitation therapy, and he and his family learned what steps might reduce the risk of another stroke. Now he is ready to resume his life and be as independent as his disability allows.

The great majority of those who have survived strokes are able to return home. But returning home may not mean returning to things exactly as they were. A certain amount of adjustment is often called for. The home itself may need to be modified or rearranged to make it as safe and accessible as possible for a person with physical or cognitive problems. In this chapter we'll look at some of those changes.

Leaving the Hospital

M ost people who survive a stroke are able to return to their homes and resume many of their activities. Others must make new living arrangements. Such adjustments are almost always a stressful event. They may be especially difficult when there is a loss of familiar surroundings, less independence, and a loss of privacy. It is no wonder that stroke survivors who are unable to return to their own homes sometimes feel confused, helpless, and even angry.

Sophie was on the phone with her brother.

"I don't think Mother should go back to her house alone, now that she's had this stroke," she said. "With Dad gone, I'd just worry all the time. She would be so far away from any of us. What do you think?"

Morris considered. "Well, I agree with you, but I don't think Mom would. And I don't know what the solution might be. I'm in an apartment. You have a house in the suburbs but also a husband and three kids. Janice lives in Florida, and you know how Mom feels about Florida! The bottom line is, none of us are really prepared to have Mom move in with us, Sophie."

"I'll check around here, and see what other people do," Sophie decided. "I'll call you back."

By the end of the next week, Sophie had located a multi-layered care facility near her home that she thought even her very independent mother might like. It would give her mother her own apartment, but nursing and other types of care would be available when necessary. She took brochures to the hospital to show her mother. She then arranged to take her mother there one day to look at it.

To Sophie's relief, her mother recognized that it was proba-bly time to move out of that big old house in the country and into something smaller and more manageable. Her mother even remarked that she was tired of all the upkeep necessary on the house. She agreed to make the move.

Several weeks later, when her mother had settled in, Sophie called her brother again.

"Mother really likes her apartment. It turns out she really likes being closer to the grandchildren. We see her more often now than we have in years. Guess what she likes even better? She loves eating down in the dining room with all the other residents! Apparently she's even found two or three who feel the same way about Florida as she does. It's worked out well. I'm happy for her."

There are ways the caregiver can help alleviate some of these feelings. If possible, involve the stroke survivor in the decision-making process. Spend time talking with the stroke survivor about the move. Discuss the positive things about the move—opportunity to build or maintain friendships, service facilities, convenience, etc. Help him become familiar with the new location before the move—through pictures or a visit. Also, spend time with the stroke survivor after the move. Provide ways to display treasured belongings in the new surroundings.

Choosing the right living arrangements for a stroke survivor is not always easy. Some stroke survivors need the continuing care available in a nursing facility. Others may find shared or enriched housing suits their needs best. Let's look at some of the options available.

Nursing Facilities

A nursing facility is the right choice for some stroke survivors. Some of these people have ongoing medical or coping problems. Some previously lived alone, without regular contact with others, and a nursing facility can give them the support they need. There are two types of facilities: skilled nursing facilities and intermediate care facilities.

Skilled nursing facilities may be called for if the stroke survivor still needs a lot of care but doesn't have someone at home to help him. These facilities offer twenty-four-hour nursing care and physical and occupational therapy. They also offer more regular doctor visits than intermediate care facilities do. They are equipped to take care of people who are bedridden as well as those who are more independent.

Skilled nursing facilities are also more costly than intermediate care ones. Stays at some institutions are partially covered by Medicare for a limited time. When you research these facilities, ask if they have Medicare certification.

Intermediate care facilities are meant for those who are more independent and have no serious medical problems. Usually they provide nursing care during the day only and twenty-four-hour supervision. They often provide social activities as well.

Residence at a nursing facility may be for the short or long term.

Sometimes a transitional stay between the hospital and home is a good idea for a bedridden person. The stroke survivor gets continuing medical attention at the nursing facility while he is gaining more strength. For a stroke survivor who was unable to participate in rehabilitation therapy while in the hospital, a nursing facility may offer an opportunity to begin therapy. Also, while the stroke survivor is in the nursing facility, the family gets some extra time to ready the house for his arrival.

Shared and Enriched Housing

Some people who have had strokes may not relish the idea of living alone again after their illness. Others may not like the idea of giving up a familiar home just because they now have trouble keeping up with the chores. Those who remain fairly independent might find shared housing a good alternative to intermediate care facilities and a way to solve these problems.

Shared housing works in two ways. For a stroke survivor who has a room to let, it can mean the renter will help with the chores and monthly household bills. For the stroke survivor who rents a room in someone else's home, it may mean he has a smaller household burden. For both parties, it can also provide the reassuring sense that another person has a general idea of their whereabouts.

Check with your place of worship or community service centers to locate reputable professional services that screen and match people for shared housing. Shared housing can be a good, logical way for two relatively compatible people to help each other remain independent.

Enriched housing may be another good choice for the relatively independent person who doesn't wish to live alone anymore. In this situation, housing is shared by three or more people, one or more of whom may be a stroke survivor. Each person has his own room, but the kitchen and living room area are shared by all. Other services may be available with enriched housing. These include laundry, some meals, or help with dressing or grooming activities. For those who qualify, enriched housing costs may be covered in part by Supplemental Security Income, a government program for older, blind, or disabled people with limited income and resources.

When Going Home Is the Right Choice

Going home poses no problem for those who experienced a so-called minor stroke and show no evidence of major disabilities. For those whose strokes were more severe, going home depends largely on four important factors.

The first is the stroke survivor's education regarding his own care. Before leaving the hospital, he should be taught all the fundamental "activities of daily living" (ADL) skills that will let him be as independent as possible. These might include dressing, grooming, and toileting skills. If necessary, he should also have learned how to compensate for sensory, perceptual, or cognitive deficits. Sometimes it's useful for the stroke survivor to stay at a rehabilitation center for intensive therapy in this area before going home. The doctor or physical therapist at the hospital can advise the stroke survivor and his family on this. Some areas don't have their own rehabilitation centers. This makes it a little harder to find the kinds of rehabilitation specialists that may be needed. Some national organizations that may provide help are listed in the Appendix (see pages 290–293).

Second, the stroke survivor should know how to monitor his own health care and be able to do so at home. He should be able to follow directions for taking any medications his doctor has prescribed, and he should be able to return reliably to his doctor's office or the hospital for scheduled checkups. He should also be prepared to practice stroke prevention, as his doctor recommends. This may mean stopping smoking or following a sensible diet. Or it may mean controlling high blood pressure or a diabetic condition. (Stroke prevention is discussed in Chapter Eight.) A person going home after a stroke should also know all the warning signs of stroke (these are listed on page 37), as should his caregivers and family members.

Third, a person going home after a stroke also needs to have a caregiver who is ready and willing to help him, as needed, with the activities of daily living. A caregiver may be a spouse, other family member, close friend, or hired nursing aide.

Fourth, the extent of the person's mobility and communication skills must also be considered. This is probably the most important factor if the stroke survivor lives alone. If these skills are poor, the

COPING WITH LIVING ALONE
IF YOU'VE HAD A STROKE

- Arrange to be called at home at least once a day.

- Develop a signal system with your neighbors that will alert them if you find yourself in trouble. This is especially important if you are unable to speak.

- Let the local fire department know of your condition. Give them your name, address, and phone number for their files. That information will help them help you in an emergency.

- Talk to your local postmaster or mail carrier about enrolling in U.S. Postal Alert. This is a program in which an identifying sticker is placed on a person's mailbox. If mail accumulates, the carrier will notify the appropriate agency or service.

stroke survivor will be extremely isolated at best and at greatly increased risk of harm because of that isolation at worst.

Returning home successfully also depends on the degree to which the home can be adapted to suit the new needs of the stroke survivor. Someone who now uses a wheelchair, for example, obviously can't return home to a walk-up apartment. Fortunately, such an extreme case is rare. In most cases, plenty can be done to make the home perfectly accessible and welcoming to one with disabilities.

In this chapter, we'll address each of these important considerations in greater depth. We'll also discuss some practical approaches to living day-to-day with a disability, from dressing to driving. We'll look at ways loved ones can learn to communicate better with stroke survivors who may be aphasic or have related problems. And we'll discuss ways both stroke survivor and family can learn to make the psychological adjustment to stroke and related disabilities. In addition, we'll address some of the community resources that might be of help.

First, let's consider some of the ways in which you, as a caregiver, might adapt your home to suit a stroke survivor's new needs and provide a safe environment.

As soon as he began to stabilize after his stroke, Richard, fifty-eight, was looking forward to going home. His thrombotic stroke had left him with a residual weakness on the right side of his body. He would go home in a wheelchair, though he still had hopes of graduating to walking with a cane in the months ahead.

Richard's wife, Inez, was eager to help make her husband's transition home as smooth as possible. With the advice of visiting nurses, she worked to adapt their home to be as comfortable for Richard as possible. Their house has two stories. The couple's bedroom had been upstairs, so the first thing Inez did was move their things into a downstairs bedroom instead. She made sure that the downstairs bathroom could accommodate a wheelchair, and she added grab bars and a night-light as well.

Looking around the first floor, Inez tried to imagine how Richard might go from room to room in a wheelchair. She tried to envision what might get in his way, then she rearranged furniture that he might bump into. She removed throw rugs that could impede his progress in a chair or that might trip him when he graduated to walking with a cane. Finally, she had a ramp built up to the kitchen door so that Richard could enter the house easily from the garage.

When Richard came home, he joked to Inez that it was easier to find things around the house now than before his stroke. He was touched by the work she had done. There were still a few things left to fix. The wires to floor lamps had to be taped down securely so a wheelchair could cross them easily, for example. Overall, things looked very good. Inez still helped Richard with some tasks, too. Visiting nurses stopped by regularly, and Inez drove Richard to his rehabilitation therapy three times a week. In the next few months, Richard gradually learned to walk again, first with a walker, and then with only a cane. That day, Richard was jubilant.

"You just wait, Inez. I'll be racing you upstairs by this time next year," Richard teased. Inez just smiled.

Adapting the Home

Going home and getting resettled after a major stroke can be a bewildering prospect to the stroke survivor and his loved ones. This is especially true if the person has severe impairments, whether physical, sensory, or perceptual. How can anyone prepare for all the frustrating or risky situations that are likely to arise in the home under those conditions?

The short answer is: No one can anticipate everything. So don't feel guilty if you can't, either. What everyone can and should do, however, is try to spot as many areas of potential difficulty for the person as possible. Still, no matter how hard you may try to avoid it, some frustration is likely to be part of the recovery process. A lot of learning on everyone's part is going to occur "on the job"— but you may discover new wellsprings of ingenuity, too!

Not everything in the home needs to be altered at once, but some things must be done before the stroke survivor comes home. It's extremely important that areas of potential danger in the home are made as safe as possible before the stroke survivor arrives. To help in this, some hospitals will send a member of the person's stroke team to the patient's home before he is discharged, if his disability is great. This specialist might be a nurse, a social worker, or a physical or occupational therapist. She knows the person's special needs and can use this knowledge to accurately assess the home environment to which the person will return. She will assess the home's accessibility, including how well the stroke survivor might get in and out of the house and move between rooms. She will also see if he can perform specific tasks in each room, such as the kitchen. Can he make transfers from bed to chair, or from chair to toilet? Can he reach a telephone? Sometimes the stroke survivor accompanies the stroke team member on this trip, which is called a "rehabilitation home visit."

The nurse, therapist, or social worker then draws up a plan and makes recommendations for the stroke survivor based on what she has observed. She might suggest certain equipment that could make performing some tasks in the home easier. Or she might suggest certain modifications for the home, such as the addition of a ramp for someone in a wheelchair or the removal of throw rugs that might trip a person in a walker. Many stroke survivors and their families find this help both useful and reassuring.

Families of stroke survivors who are not severely disabled may be asked to make an assessment of their home on their own. The stroke team will use that information to make an "off-site" evaluation.

It may also be a good idea for those who have been severely disabled by their strokes to "try out" life back at home a few times before being discharged from the hospital. The visits usually last one to two days. During this time the patient gets the chance to practice what he has been learning in rehab and to get a sense of what adjustments he may still need to make. His family gets the chance to adjust its routines and to try caregiving. After they see how it goes, the family may still need to learn a bit more before the loved one comes home to stay. This trial period gives everyone the opportunity to address any last-minute difficulties. Afterward, both the stroke survivor and the family can assess the experience with the appropriate member or members of the stroke team and receive help or advice as needed. These visits are called "therapeutic home passes."

Accessibility

Accessibility allows a person to get around and do things as independently and safely as possible, without being blocked by physical barriers. A barrier might be as "minor" as the three steps leading up to the door of a popular gardening store. To a gardener in a wheelchair, that "minor" barrier is literally insurmountable. A barrier might also be high kitchen shelves that put a colander out of reach. Accessibility—in the home, in public places, and at work —generally requires making some adjustments in those places to accommodate people who are disabled. Fortunately, many of these adjustments are inexpensive and easy to make. More and more new buildings are being designed with "universal access" in mind. That is, they are automatically accessible to the able-bodied and disabled alike. And now, for the majority of businesses, providing access in some measure is the law, even in older buildings.

In 1991 the federal government passed the Americans with Disabilities Act. This act benefits not only people who can't walk, but also those who are blind or deaf or have mental disabilities. Title III of the act, which became effective early in 1992, addressed the problem of access. It requires all businesses that provide services to the public to remove physical barriers that may prevent a person who is disabled from using those services. These businesses include everything from motels to restaurants, schools to senior centers. (The act does make a distinction between small businesses with limited financial resources and large corporations or public institutions.) Accommodations could be as elaborate as adding an elevator and automatic doors in a large auditorium. Or they could be as simple as reserving advantageous parking spaces in a grocery store lot for drivers who are disabled. Fulfilling the requirement might even be as simple as making a service employee available to procure items that a person with a disability can't reach or get by himself. (This is one solution to our gardener's dilemma in the previous paragraph.)

Evaluating the Home

How can you make your home more accessible to those with disabilities? This job is usually made easier with advice from the stroke team member who has visited your home. You may have to make modifications to the home in general or to specific rooms. You may need to add special equipment or even change the physical layout of the home itself. Each of these changes can make getting around the home easier and safer.

Let's take a look at some of the general adaptations that you may wish to consider. Let's start with the overall layout of the home and then do room-by-room assessments. As you read this section, you may want to draw up a couple of lists of the things that need to be adjusted in your own home. The first list should describe what jobs must be done immediately. It should include changes that need to be made for safety reasons and those that would greatly improve the person's initial mobility and independence. You may also include on this list jobs that are relatively simple. A second list might describe adaptations that will improve a disabled person's life at home but aren't absolutely necessary. These jobs might take more planning and time to execute.

Approaching the Home

Can the person who is disabled approach the house with relative ease? If she is in a wheelchair, consider the problem of stairs, steep driveways, broken sidewalks, and narrow paths that may lead from the driveway to the door. Let's look at some specific areas to consider in your assessment.

Slope. A steep slope in the driveway or at the entrance to the home can make maneuvering a wheelchair very difficult, if not impossible. If ramps are called for, they should not be too steep. The recommended slope for a ramp is no more than a one-foot rise for every twelve feet of ramp. That equals an 8.3 percent grade, or a 4- to 5-degree angle. In some cases, a chairlift may work better than a ramp.

Parking. How close can the car be parked to the house? If there is a garage, will the person who is disabled have room to open the door adequately to get out and maneuver? If there isn't a garage, what kind of terrain will the stroke survivor have to cross to reach the house?

Walkways, Sidewalks, and Driveways. Consider the surface and width of the pathway and its connection to ramps, doorways, platforms, etc. What are the surfaces like? A nonskid surface is the most desirable. A surface that is too rough or broken—such as a dirt path or a path made of flagstones—can make maneuvering a wheelchair nearly impossible. A very smooth surface, such as smooth concrete, can also be trouble in some cases. When such a surface gets wet, slipping and skidding often result—a potentially dangerous situation. Would the stroke survivor have to cross a lawn to get from the driveway to the door? Lawns can be fairly easy to get across if the grass is short and dry, but difficult if the grass is long or wet.

Measure the width of the pathways. Would they accommodate a wheelchair or walker? Pay attention also to those places where two types of surfaces join. For example, if a ramp is installed between the front door and the walkway that leads to it, be sure the person can move easily from one to the other. A smooth surface should be maintained between the two so that it will be easy to get the wheelchair or walker over that spot.

Lighting. This is an important consideration both inside and outside the home. Adequate lighting is a must along walkways, on ramps, and in the garage so it's easy to see edges and potential trouble spots in the path.

Handrails and Guardrails. Sturdy handrails should extend along all ramps and up stairs at a comfortable level. If the person who will be using the handrail has hemiplegia (paralysis on one side of the body), be sure to consider which side she favors before you install the handrail. A handrail that is rounded on top and has grooves on the side may be more comfortable to grasp than one that has square edges and straight sides. Install a lower guardrail on ramps to prevent the wheelchair from accidentally slipping under the handrail and over the ramp edge.

Entrance. The traditional front door, which often has steps leading up to it, may not be the most convenient entrance for a person who is disabled. The back door, a side door, or the door from the garage may be preferable. If a long ramp or lift is needed, a side door might provide more room to set up the arrangement. Consider all the entrances to your home and choose the one that will be easiest to modify. Consider how the stroke survivor will reach that door. Be sure that the door is wide enough to accommodate any special equipment, such as a wheelchair. Removing the doorsill may make getting over the entrance a little easier.

Inside the Home

An assessment of the inside of the home should begin with the general layout of the rooms and their accessibility. After that, look at the kinds of furniture and other items found in the home. Are there items that may present a safety hazard or be a source of frustration to the person who is disabled? You may need to move some items to a different place or remove them altogether. You may need to add other safety features as well. Let's look at some specifics.

Stairs. Can the person who is disabled get up and down the stairs within the home? Would sturdy handrails be enough to make them negotiable? If not, would it be possible to install an electric lift?

If the person will be living on the first floor only, does he have all the accommodations he needs to make this area comfortable and acceptable to him? Are the kitchen, his bedroom, bathroom, dining room, and family or living room all accessible on this level? They need to be.

GETTING AROUND SAFELY IN THE HOME IF YOU'VE HAD A STROKE

Fit your walker or cane with rubber tips, which grip the floor more securely.

If you use crutches, clean the tips regularly with steel wool or other abrasive.

Choose shoes with low, strong, solid heels. Choose slip-proof rubber heels.

Avoid slippery waxed floors. If your floors must be waxed, use a skid-proof type of wax or change to a waxless linoleum flooring.

Remove throw rugs from the home if possible; they cause slips and trips. If you must have them, use extra precautions. Secure them to the floor around all edges with carpet tape or nails. Wall-to-wall carpeting is okay if the pile is short. Avoid shag rugs, which are hard to maneuver across.

Will the stroke survivor be using more than one floor in the home? If so he will need to have a telephone, fire extinguisher, and smoke detectors on every floor as a sensible safety precaution. (We'll discuss safety requirements more fully on page 177.)

Doorways. If doorways have to be wide enough to accommodate a wheelchair, measure them ahead of time. It's possible to buy a device that reduces chair width if necessary (ask at the business where you acquired the chair). Removing a door can also "add" width to the space.

Doors can also be difficult for some people to open. Consider changing the kind of door handle to one that is easier to manipulate, or remove the door altogether. Be sure that any doorsills are manageable, especially if they lie between rooms with two different kinds of flooring.

Flooring. Some kinds of flooring are easier to manage than others. Nonskid surfaces are safest for everyone. Don't wax floors—it makes them dangerously slippery.

Rugs can be a problem. Throw rugs can trip people; it's best to remove them unless you can solidly secure them around all edges and keep them from slipping as well. If they are too bulky or sit too high on the floor, they can be more trouble than they are worth. Wall-to-wall carpeting can be okay if it is of a short pile or indoor/outdoor type. It is very difficult to maneuver wheelchairs, canes, or walkers over deep-pile rugs, such as shag rugs. In fact, deep-pile rugs are not appropriate for anyone who has any trouble walking.

Furniture. We'll get to specifics about furniture in a moment, when we go through the home room by room. For now, be sure that there is plenty of space around tables, sofas, and other furniture. This allows a person with disabilities to navigate more easily through rooms. Does any of the furniture have low, sharp angles that might catch on someone's leg or equipment? That sort of furniture should be moved as far out of the way as possible. Those who are in wheelchairs or who can't reach for things easily may need shelves, sinks, and the like lowered, too.

Lighting and Mirrors. Inadequate lighting can indeed present a barrier to the person who is disabled. Hallways, rooms, and closets should be well lit. The person should be able to manipulate the light switches for himself, including one for a reading lamp in the bedroom. For those with a sensory deficit, a night-light in the bedroom, perhaps accompanied by soft music from the radio, can help make the dark seem less isolating. A night-light in the bathroom may be a good idea also.

Adjustable mirrors that can be brought close from a wall mounting may be ideal for some. The best place for a mirror depends on the individual person. So try to find out from him what might be best, or observe him closely to see what seems to work for him.

Extension Cords. Cables, cords, or exposed wires should be run as much as possible along the baseboards of walls and covered with electrical tape. Leaving loose cords from lamps, computers, toasters, or other appliances invites accidents. Not only can cords trip people, but they can pull down and break expensive household equipment. They can even cause sparks that can lead to a fire. Get them out of the way as soon as possible!

Safety Equipment. In an emergency, speed counts. Getting to a phone or putting out a fire could mean the difference between life and death. In assessing the home, give a lot of attention to safety features that might improve the odds in case of emergency. If the person who is disabled lives in a multilevel home, telephones, smoke detectors, and fire extinguishers should be installed on every floor to which she has access.

How many telephones are in the house, and where are they located? Consider adding extensions to every room, or at least to those in which the person who is disabled spends most of her time. Be sure to keep important emergency numbers next to, if not taped to, every phone. If your phones allow you to preset some numbers, be sure to set them up so the stroke survivor can use them easily.

Where are the fire extinguishers located? Keep a fire extinguisher in the kitchen, readily accessible to the stove and easy to use. Be sure everyone in the house knows how to use it properly, and remember to have it tested or replaced periodically, as required.

Smoke detectors should also be strategically located in the home, including in the kitchen and bedroom areas. Smoke detectors save lives. Be sure yours are tested regularly, and replace the batteries regularly.

Adapting Specific Rooms
The general information given above applies to every room in the home. Let's look at some suggestions for adapting specific rooms that may need some special care. (Transfers will be discussed later, on pages 188–195.)

Bedroom. A few special considerations should be made for those who are confined to bed, and also for anyone who is expected to spend a lot of time initially in the bedroom. It may be a good idea to lower the bed to make transfers from bed to wheelchair easier, if that will be necessary. In this case, there also should be enough space between the bed and the wall to accommodate the wheel-chair.

A portable bedside toilet may be a good idea, especially if the stroke survivor is bedridden or if he needs to make frequent trips to the bathroom in the night.

The person who has had a stroke should have a bedside table for any items he may need, such as tissues, other toiletries, and drink-ing water. A small bell is handy to summon family members. A comfortable reading lamp is a good idea. The stroke survivor should be able to work the switch.

Special arrangements may be needed if the person has neglect of a side (ignores half of his visual field and/or one side of his body). When there are visitors, keep some items, such as water or tissues, on the neglected side. The visitors can remind him of the location of the items so he can practice using his neglected side to get to them. At night or when the stroke survivor is alone, however, these items should all be available to him from his unimpaired side.

Bathroom. The first consideration is to make it as easy as possible for the person who is disabled to get through the house to the bathroom. First, make sure that the distance involved between any commonly used room and the bathroom is not too great. Then, move unnecessary furniture or equipment out of the way. Finally, be sure there is adequate lighting.

The bathroom is a complicated place, with several functions and a lot of equipment vying for space. It is a common site for accidents for anyone, but can perhaps be especially hazardous to those with disabilities. With a little attention to detail, however, many of the difficulties the bathroom may present can be overcome.

Because bathrooms are frequently so small, their layouts can be particularly important to people with disabilities. Using a wheel-chair or other equipment in the same small space that includes a toilet, shower or bathtub, and sink presents some special problems. First, there needs to be adequate space for a wheelchair. Some people will need to do a transfer in the bathroom. A wheelchair must be parked alongside of whatever the person is being transferred

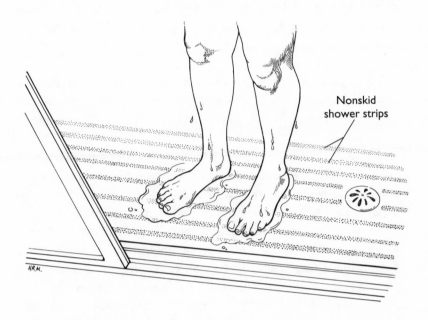

Nonskid
shower strips

A nonskid surface on the shower floor will help prevent slips and falls.

to—in this case, a toilet, tub, or shower. Know the dimensions of
the wheelchair and measure the bathroom for these tasks.

Grab bars in the bathroom, where slips and falls are common,
are a good idea for almost everyone. But for anyone who is already
unsteady, they are extremely important. Horizontal grab bars might
be useful along the wall on either side of the toilet. Vertical and
horizontal bars should also be installed in the tub and shower. The
exact placement depends on the arrangement of your bathroom.
Horizontal grab bars are for pushing up from, while vertical grab
bars are for pulling on. Be sure they are installed in a very secure,
permanent manner.

Transfers to and from a toilet may be made easier for some if the
toilet seat is adapted to be higher than usual. You may buy devices
for this purpose at a medical supply store.

Aside from grab bars, other adaptations can be made to the tub
or shower in the home. Use a rubber mat or a nonskid surface on
the bottom of the tub or shower stall. Putting a stool or straight-
backed chair in the bathtub or shower allows the bather to sit

179

rather than stand for a shower. The stool or chair should have rubber-tipped legs to prevent sliding. Hand-held shower heads make bathing easier. If a shower stall is to be used, make sure the bather can get over the sill between the shower and the floor.

Faucets should be made easy to maneuver. Small handles may prove awkward for some. You may want to replace these with large wing-type handles that can be moved using the wrist or arm instead of the hand.

The sink area may need some renovation. Someone in a wheel-chair may not be able to get close enough to wash her hands or face if there is a cupboard underneath, blocking her knees. Some sink designs, such as a pedestal base, do allow a closer approach.

Those who have sensory deficits must be particularly careful not to use water that is too hot or to bump against hot water pipes. Serious burns may result. To be safe, cover any exposed hot water pipes. (Your local hardware store will show you what works best.) Always turn on the cool water tap first. Then slowly add water from the hot tap after that. Similarly, always turn off the hot water tap before the cool water tap. It is best to bathe in lukewarm water.

A number of devices can help make grooming simpler. Soap on a rope, hung around the neck, keeps soap close at hand during showering. It never slips to the floor, where it could be hard to reach. Or soap might be enclosed in a washcloth pouch or mitt—it's easier to handle and helps the stroke survivor use two related items at once. (If washcloths are hard on delicate skin, try using soft brushes instead.) Suction pads with hooks in the tub or shower can hold some toiletry articles (such as nailbrushes) in handy, secure places.

Many grooming articles, including hairbrushes, toothbrushes, and lotion bottles, can be hard to hold after a stroke. It can help to wrap the handles of these items in a thick spongy material, which makes them easier to grasp. These everyday articles should be arranged in the bathroom in a convenient, accessible way. They shouldn't be stored in hard-to-reach places, such as under the sink or in a crowded medicine chest.

Ruben had had a stroke about six months before and now used a wheelchair. Adjusting to the chair had been difficult for him. Eventually he had mastered moving from bed to chair and was much more independent.

Before his stroke, Ruben had been everyone's favorite uncle, sharing stories, teasing and playing with the kids, and flattering the grandmas. But since his stroke, Ruben had become more subdued. He seemed uncertain, and he was less fun-loving than he had been. It seemed that he just didn't care as much as he had about his personal grooming and cleanliness. That was what really bothered his family and friends the most.

Finally, Ruben's wife, Luna, spoke to him about this problem and asked if there was anything she could do for him.

"I hate having to ask you all the time for help to do anything in the bathroom," Ruben said. "I'd almost just rather not do it than have to ask all the time!"

Luna could see that her husband was frustrated by this lack of privacy. She said she would see whether the bathroom could be fixed somehow so he could get to whatever he needed, himself.

Luna called the occupational therapist who had worked with her husband at the hospital and asked her what might help. She was relieved to find that a number of simple changes could be made that could make all the difference to her husband.

With the help of a carpenter and instructions from the therapist, the bathroom was adapted to accommodate Ruben in his wheelchair. First, they removed the existing sink, which had built-in cabinets below it. They put in a pedestal-style sink that Ruben could put his knees underneath. He could get much closer to the sink that way. Then they installed grab bars around the toilet, making transfers much easier.

Finally, they adapted the tub. First they added grab bars there, too. Then they put in a flexible shower head that allowed Ruben to hold it in one hand and direct the spray wherever he wanted it. Luna bought a small, sturdy stool with rubber-tipped feet that could sit in the tub securely. Luna still needs to help Ruben get into and out of the tub safely, but now he is on his own otherwise.

These changes made a world of difference to Ruben. He has shown a greater interest in grooming. He feels better about himself and seems more interested in his friends and family. Just the other day he told one of his famous stories about "the good ole days" when he got his first car.

Living Room. Many of the points to remember when assessing the accessibility of the living room have already been discussed. Carpeting should be close-cropped. Throw rugs should be eliminated or secured along all edges to the floor, using carpet tape or nails. The room should be well lit.

Furniture should not crowd the area. There should be plenty of room for the person who is disabled to maneuver comfortably in. In addition, the furniture should all be raised to wheelchair height, if necessary. This allows for easier transfers. Wooden blocks can do the trick here. So can firm cushions added to chair seats.

Kitchen. The kitchen, like the bath, is a busy room in which a lot can go wrong. Make safety in this room a high priority. Here are some things to think about as you go.

Be sure the room and the work surfaces in the room are well lit. All light switches should be within the reach of the person who is disabled.

If possible, select a stove that has the controls in front, rather than at the back of the stove. It is best if the front and back burners are staggered slightly, too, so the cook doesn't have to reach over a hot area to stir something in back. If the stroke survivor can't reach the stove safely, he can use a hot plate on the kitchen table instead.

Turning off the oven and burners as soon as you are finished is always a good idea. A person who is disabled may want to use a timer to help remind him to do so. Remind the person to always turn pan handles in, away from the edge of the stove. This reduces the likelihood of being burned by spilled food that is still cooking. Select pans with handles that don't conduct heat. Have mesh screens handy for covering fry pans to prevent splattering and grease burns.

Keep curtains, blinds, paper towels, and dish towels—or anything that could catch fire—away from the stove.

Many of the precautions that make sense for a bathroom sink make sense for a kitchen sink, too. Be careful of hot water. Cover any exposed hot water pipes. Turn on the cool tap first, and then slowly add water from the hot tap to reach the desired water temperature. Buy faucets that can be turned on and off with the wrists or arms rather than the hands, if necessary. Don't use any electrical appliances near water.

Keep a nonskid rubber mat in front of the sink to help prevent slips. And speaking of slipping, a reminder: Don't wax the kitchen linoleum, even if it has always been waxed. It will make the floor dangerously slippery, and "pretty" just isn't worth the risk. (Besides, no-wax linoleum is available today.)

Remind family members to clean up all spills quickly. Whether wet or dry, spills cause falls. A long-handled mop or broom and a long-handled dustpan make it possible to do the job while sitting or standing.

There are a number of ways to make the kitchen cupboards and counters more accessible. Counters, the sink, cupboard space, and tables all should be at the same acceptable height. The table or some counter space should also have leg room underneath, so a person can slide in as close as possible to the work surface. (It helps if the sink can be arranged this way, too.)

The items that the person who is disabled will need regularly in the kitchen should be arranged in cupboards or shelves that fall within his reach. Try to avoid storing anything in places where someone will have to bend over or reach up to get them, or have to open or close doors. Long-handled reachers or tongs can help people securely grasp some small, light things that otherwise remain out of reach. Utility carts on casters or wheels can be useful, too. Some people find them helpful for kitchen storage. Others use them while cooking to hold ingredients collected beforehand from the refrigerator, cupboards, and counters. This saves them energy because they don't have to go back and forth in the kitchen as they cook.

Check to see where electrical outlets fall on counters. Can the person who is disabled easily reach one in order to plug in an

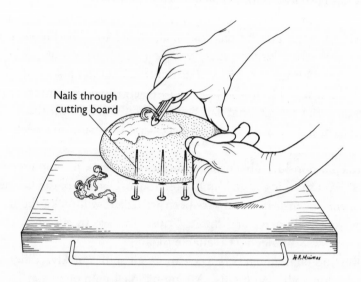

Nails through
cutting board

A special cutting board can make food preparation much easier.

appliance? If not, it may make sense to move an outlet up to counter level.

Separate sharp utensils and tools from the others in drawers. Keep knives in a covered rack.

Be sure the person who is disabled wears nonflammable clothing in the kitchen. Clothing that is excessively loose or has ruffles could get caught in an appliance or catch fire from the stovetop. Keep long nonflammable kitchen mitts and potholders nearby to protect hands and forearms. Avoid plastic aprons, which may melt if hot oil splashes on them or they accidentally come in contact with a hot surface such as the edge of the oven door.

Consider having a special cutting board made if the person who is disabled will be doing much cooking. A regular cutting board, modified with a few short nails that poke up from the bottom, can make the job much easier. Food, such as potatoes, can be impaled on the spikes and then carefully cut up or peeled using one hand.

Here are some extra tips to make working in the kitchen a good experience. Remind the cook with disabilities to keep his hands dry at all times; it's easier to drop things if one's hands are wet or oily. Remind him also to move slowly and carefully as he works. If he has any sensory deficit in his hands or arms, consult the occupational therapist for more kitchen precautions.

While she was in the hospital after her stroke, Emily kept saying that all she wanted to do was go home and fix her family and friends a big meal. She loved to cook, and she was very good at it. But her stroke had left her with weakness on her right side. She was able to walk with the help of a cane. When she returned home, she found that some kitchen jobs that she used to love had become, well, chores.

"What am I going to do, girl?" she asked her best friend, Melanie, one day in exasperation. "I can't chop anything without the board sliding all around the table. I can't hold onto it and chop at the same time. And I have to use this old cane even when I only need to cross the room for a spice or something I forgot to put into the recipe. I could go on. I'm not having fun with this anymore."

Melanie went shopping the next day. She returned to Emily's kitchen with a bag full of gadgets she thought might help keep Emily cooking. In the bag was a new, heavy chopping board with three little nails poking up randomly through the bottom. "I thought you could stick the food on the nails to hold them while you chop," Melanie said. Emily was delighted.

"I brought you some other stuff, too, Emily," Melanie said, continuing to pull items from the sack. "Here's a set of plastic mixing bowls with suction cups on the bottom so they don't slide when you're stirring. Neat, huh? I could use some of those! Here's a rubber mat to put in front of the sink so you won't slip if it gets wet there. And here's a long-handled grabber so you can pull down little stuff that's otherwise out of reach in your cabinets. I like to call this one 'Jaws.' Well, what do you think?"

"I think you're the greatest, Melanie," Emily said. "You and that dear man who is my husband. Ernest has also heard me complaining about my kitchen. Look at this! He brought this desk in here this morning so I can sit down to do some of my prep work. See, it's lower than the counter and I can scoot a chair in underneath, too. And he got me this utility cart. I can roll it around the kitchen once and put everything in it that I'm going to need to make dinner or whatever. I don't have to get up and down anymore! I can keep my favorite tools in it, too. They're always handy. And you know what else? Ernest is helping me cook now. And I really enjoy that. He does, too."

"That's great, Emily."

"Thank you so much, Melanie," Emily said. "I feel inspired again. Maybe fish tonight. Will you stay for dinner?"

7
Living
with a Disability

A stroke is likely to leave behind a variety of problems that may range from mild to severe. The ability to move, see, speak, and understand others can all be compromised by a stroke. All of these problems may require changes in behavior or movement to compensate. Coping with this reality can be very hard, and a certain amount of anxiety is normal for both the person who has had a stroke and his loved ones. Coping with the changes stroke may bring is important. In this chapter, we'll look at ways to help make that process easier for everyone. We'll discuss the variety of challenges this new situation presents and show how they might be met successfully.

An occupational therapist may be able to help you devise new skills to accomplish old tasks. Family and friends need to show their patience and support now, too. And, as we'll see, help is available from many sources.

Coping with the Activities of Daily Living (ADLs) —Tips for the Person Who Is Disabled

Although it's hard to do at times, remember that you are a stroke survivor. What you are learning is essentially new, and it will take time to master. What used to take a minute and a half to do or say may now take much longer. It may require more thought and effort as well. Frustration can run high. Work slowly, and be generous with yourself if you make a mistake—or even a lot of mistakes! People who have had a stroke very commonly mix up a sequence of steps when they try to accomplish a task, or are unable to coordinate their movements well. They may also try to rush into an activity that was familiar to them prior to their stroke.

While you're relearning skills, you may need reminders to start tasks slowly. It's easiest to follow instructions that are simple, listed one step at a time. Relax and keep a positive outlook. You may have to do a task many times before you learn it.

In this section, we'll look at some of the more common activities of daily living, or ADLs, and suggest some alternative approaches to and helpful aids for those familiar skills.

Transfers

A transfer is a move from one location to another. Moving from a chair to your bed, or from a wheelchair to a toilet, bathtub, or car are all examples of transfers. You may use a **sliding board** to help with transfers. A nurse, physical therapist, or occupational therapist should teach you the proper way to make transfers. Be sure to follow her directions. The tips below may help you review the necessary steps.

Four rules are necessary for safe transfers:

1. The surface you're transferring to and the surface you're transferring from should be the same height.
2. The two surfaces should be as close together as possible.
3. You should lead with your stronger side unless your therapist tells you otherwise.
4. Put on your shoes and braces (if prescribed) before any transfer, unless you're going to take a bath or shower. If your affected arm is limp, you can put it in a sling before moving.

Some of these suggestions for transfers may not work for you. Use those that are most suited to your own needs.

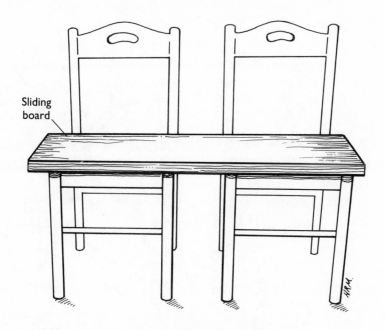

Sliding
board

A sliding board is often used in doing transfers.

Standing and Sitting Transfers

Standing and sitting are the two basic kinds of transfers. Here are some suggestions.

Stroke survivors who are paralyzed or weak on one side usually have enough strength in one or both legs to support their weight, so they can do a standing transfer. Doing a standing transfer (moving from sitting to standing, then sitting again) by yourself requires balance and arm strength, but with practice you'll improve and will need less and less help. Get only the help you need—the less help you get, the faster you'll improve. Don't take unnecessary chances, though.

You will need to do a sitting transfer if both your legs are paralyzed, or if you're unable to help with the transfer. If this is your situation, ask your therapist about using a sliding board.

Other suggestions:

- Wear a firm leather belt around your waist. If you need help, a helper can grab it.

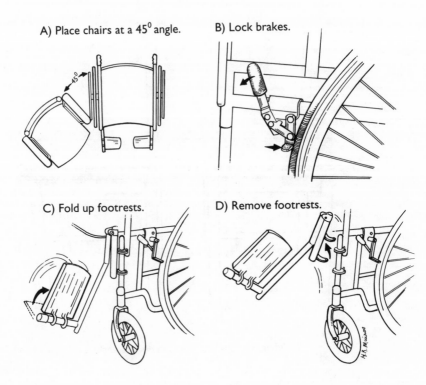

A) Place chairs at a 45° angle.

B) Lock brakes.

C) Fold up footrests.

D) Remove footrests.

Positioning the wheelchair correctly is very important when doing a transfer.

- If you use a wheelchair:
  1. If the armrests are not removable, position your wheelchair at a 45-degree angle to the other sur-face. If the armrests are removable, position the chair beside the other surface.
  2. Lock the brakes on the wheelchair.
  3. Remove the footrests.
- If you use a sliding board, rest it securely on both surfaces.

To do a standing transfer without another person's help:

1. Move to the edge of the bed or chair and sit with your feet touching the floor.
2. Place your feet so that the stronger foot is in front of your weaker foot.

3. Bend forward, push down on the bed or the chair's armrest, and stand up. If you're moving from or to a wheelchair, be sure the brakes are locked.
4. Turn your body so your back is to the front of the seat you're transferring to and bend forward slightly. After that, lower yourself to a sitting position by holding onto the arms of the chair.

To do a sitting transfer without another person's help:

1. Move to the side of your bed or chair and sit with your feet touching the floor.
2. Remove the armrests from your wheelchair.
3. Lean forward and do short push-ups to shift your hips and point them toward the surface you want to move to.
4. While leaning forward, do another series of push-ups to lift yourself out of the chair and onto the other surface.
5. As you shift, adjust the position of your legs.
6. Replace the armrests on your wheelchair and use them to bring yourself to an upright, sitting position.

Ben had just been admitted to the rehabilitation center. He had come from the hospital, where he had stabilized after having a major stroke. His stroke had paralyzed his left side, and he was here to get some intensive rehabilitation and maximize his independence. The first thing he would learn, his therapists told him, would be to make a successful independent seated transfer.

Like to a bus? Ben wondered. Isn't that a little premature? But it turned out that a bus transfer wasn't what his therapists had in mind at all. They wanted him to learn how to move from his bed to a wheelchair, and from a wheelchair to any other seated position, and back. Ben had already been working on increasing his arm strength while still in the hospital. He felt ready to try this new experience and to see what would happen.

Cynthia, the occupational therapy specialist, asked Ben to sit up in bed and swing his feet over the side, near his wheelchair. The wheelchair had been pulled up alongside the bed.

Ben did as he was asked. His feet brushed the floor as he sat on the side of the bed. "Good!" Cynthia said.

Ben laughed. "That took me weeks to learn, I want you to know," he said, smiling.

Next, Cynthia told Ben to lean over and lift up the armrests on his wheelchair. This Ben found harder, because he felt less securely balanced when he bent forward. He went very slowly. Cynthia, who was watching everything he did, approved of this. "Great!" she said. "I have put a sliding board between the bed and the chair, because you're going to use that to get into the wheelchair."

Cynthia sat on the empty bed across the room to show Ben what she wanted him to do next. "OK, are you sure the brakes are on on the chair? They are? Good. Now you have to use your arms and do short little push-ups—like this, see—to move your hips into position for getting into the wheelchair. You kind of pivot your hips onto the board and scoot across. . . . You try it, Ben."

Ben did, but he lurched unsteadily at first and had to attempt it several times. "Whew, it's tiring!" he admitted.

"Take your time. It is tiring, especially at first, I know," Cynthia said. "But we're just starting. We'll take all the time we need."

After a short break, the pair continued. "OK, Ben, now lean forward some more, and do some more push-ups to move off the bed and onto the chair, using the board . . . not too fast. . . . That's good! Don't forget to bring your legs along! They need to be adjusted as you go. . . . That's right. That looks very good. Congratulations!"

"I did it!" Ben was very pleased with his success.

He practiced making transfers repeatedly in the following weeks. He also learned to do a number of other activities. He left the rehab center a few weeks later with a very positive feeling about his many new skills and capabilities.

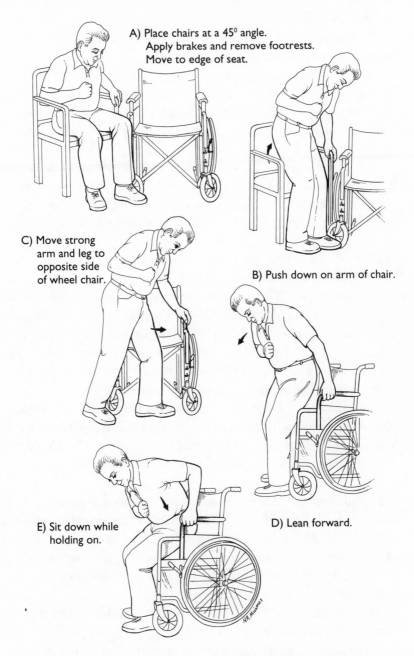

A) Place chairs at a 45⁰ angle.
   Apply brakes and remove footrests.
   Move to edge of seat.

B) Push down on arm of chair.

C) Move strong arm and leg to opposite side of wheel chair.

D) Lean forward.

E) Sit down while holding on.

Doing a standing transfer from a chair to a wheelchair involves several steps.

193

Special Transfers

Car. Transfers to and from a car are usually easier if you use the front seat—you have more space to work with since the front seat is usually wider. The first step is to bring your wheelchair as close to the car as possible and angle the chair slightly. Roll down the car window and use the door as a support. If you stand to transfer, support yourself on the door, turn, and sit down. If you're getting into a car, sit sideways and then swing your legs into the car.

When you're getting out of a car, pivot on your seat and swing your legs outside the car before you stand. Then, using the car door to brace yourself, turn and get into the wheelchair. If you sit to transfer, use a sliding board to make your transfer easier.

Toilet. A transfer to the toilet may present special problems because space is usually limited and the arrangement of most bathrooms is cramped. To do a sitting transfer, put your wheelchair as close to the toilet as you can. Installing grab bars at a 45-degree angle on your stronger side will help you sit and stand. Since the standard toilet seat is only 16 inches high, you may need to install a raised toilet seat or rely on someone to help you.

If you stand up to transfer, loosen your clothing when you're out of the wheelchair. Don't let go of the grab bars—hold on to them the whole time you're transferring. If you sit to transfer, having a removable armrest on your wheelchair is helpful. Toilet paper should be within easy reach of your stronger hand.

Tub and Shower. Before you do a transfer from a wheelchair to a shower, have vertical and horizontal grab bars installed in the shower. Place a rubber mat on the bottom of the shower. Put a stool or straight-backed chair in the shower so you can sit rather than stand. Sitting while bathing will save you a lot of energy. It's a necessary adaptation for those who use a wheelchair. The stool or chair should be the same height as your wheelchair and should have rubber-tipped legs to prevent sliding.

Arrange your wheelchair in the same direction as the stool or chair. Follow the instructions for a standing or sitting transfer given on pages 188–193. The same principle can be applied to doing a transfer from a wheelchair to a bathtub or from a chair to a tub or shower.

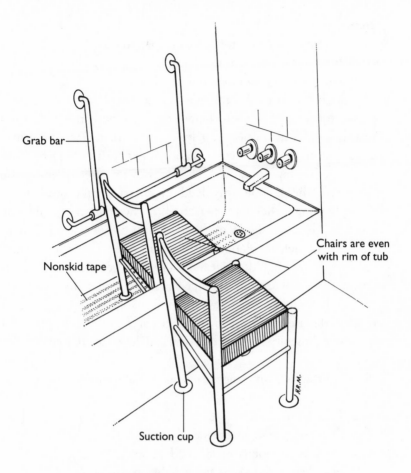

Grab bar

Nonskid tape

Chairs are even with rim of tub

Suction cup

Having two chairs side by side with one in the tub makes getting in and out of the tub a little easier.

If you use a tub rather than a shower stall, take great care when moving in and out. Place a rubber mat on the bottom of the tub. Step into the tub with your weaker side first, and step out leading with your stronger side. Be sure that both your stronger arm and the tub edge are dry as you make these moves so you can get a secure grip. When getting out of the tub, it's a good idea to leave the water in until you are out. The buoyancy of the water helps you lift yourself up.

A strong person might also help you in and out of the tub. But use extreme caution if you try this method! Both of you can easily fall and be injured. Getting out of a tub is harder than getting in.

Eating

Eating can pose problems for some people after a stroke. They may lack feeling in their mouth, or on one side of their mouth, making chewing and swallowing more difficult. If you have such a problem, or if you choke on food sometimes, consult with your doctor. He may suggest a rehabilitation therapist to help with the mechanics of eating and a nutritionist to help with your diet. Treatment may include training in breath control and proper positioning while you are eating. Therapy may involve exercises for strengthening the tongue and the muscles involved in chewing and swallowing. When planning a diet for a person with chewing and swallowing difficulties, the consistency of the food must be considered. Thickened liquids, such as blended drinks, are often easier to tolerate than thin, watery liquids. Soft foods may also be tolerated in small amounts. The diet section that appears in the Appendix (see pages 279–289) is included for use by stroke survivors and others without special dietary needs. If you are a stroke survivor with chewing and swallowing difficulties, a nutritionist can help decide what foods are best for you.

Some of the following suggestions may make eating easier.

- Take small bites.
- Chew on the stronger side of your mouth.
- Clear your mouth of all food between bites. Otherwise, bits of food may get caught on the weak side of your mouth. (Check for this with your finger or a small mirror, and remove any food with your tongue or fingers.)
- Some foods are easier to eat than others. Soft foods, for example, are easier to eat than liquids for some people. You may wish to use a blender to make the foods you like easier to swallow. Or consult a dietitian, who can recommend easy-to-swallow foods that are nutritious. (To find a dietitian, consult your hospital or local health department.)

Fortunately, most people do return eventually to a regular diet after their strokes. The American Heart Association recommends a diet that is well balanced and low in fat and cholesterol.

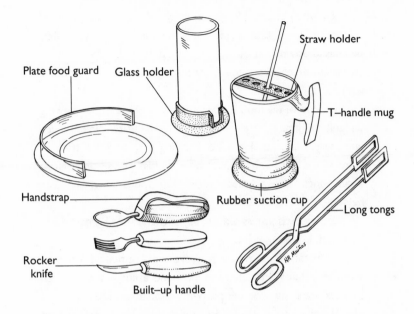

Many special tools are available to make eating a little easier.

Using forks, knives, and spoons requires extremely fine hand coordination. After a stroke, many people find it difficult to get the hang of using utensils again. Patience and practice are key to relearning the skills involved.

There are many special utensils designed to make eating easier. A "rocker knife," which cuts meat with a minimum of hand movement, is available through specialty stores. Suction cups placed on the bottom of dishes can help prevent them from sliding around on the table. A damp dish towel placed underneath the plate can also serve this purpose. A plastic rim around a dinner plate can help a one-handed individual push food onto a fork or spoon more easily. Lazy Susan table organizers can put salt, pepper, condiments, and extra napkins within close range. An occupational therapist can suggest other useful tools as well.

After his stroke, Jim had a few frustrating deficits to contend with, but none that bothered him so much as his new difficulties eating. Because of weakness on his right side, he found he couldn't use both hands in the natural, unconscious way he was

197

used to when eating. He quickly realized that without a hand to secure it, his plate would scoot around on the table while he chased down a bit of food. He couldn't hold his plate to cut anything—it always slipped. And forget peas! They were a nightmare.

One side of his mouth was numb, too. That made chewing difficult for Jim. Several times he had started to choke, which was scary. Now he chewed everything very well and tried to keep all the food in his mouth over on his "good" side before swallowing. He was eating more soft foods now, and that helped.

Mealtime was just as exhausting as the rest of his day, these days. It didn't seem right.

Fortunately, these problems were easily remedied. Through a special catalog, Mae, Jim's wife, found a number of kitchen gadgets made just for people with disabilities. She got Jim a special knife that rocked back and forth to cut, rather than requiring separate slicing movements. She got Jim a plate with a suction bottom, so it wouldn't slip, and a rubber rim, so he could push food up against it and catch it on his utensils. She also got him eating utensils with bulky foam-rubber handles that were easier to grip with a weak hand.

Because of weakness and numbness on the right side of his face, Jim sometimes had a little trouble chewing and swallowing some foods, too. Even when Mae tried to get him to drink thin soups, Jim just couldn't seem to manage. Mae decided to call Mary Jane, the nutritionist who had helped Jim at the hospital. Mary Jane was very helpful. She prepared a list of soft foods that Jim should eat and a list of foods to avoid. Mae was surprised to learn that, for Jim, soft foods were actually easier to swallow than liquefied ones. Mary Jane worked out an eating plan for Jim and gave Mae a copy of it. The soft foods that were best for Jim were incorporated into a balanced daily diet developed just for him. Now Mae is learning a new way of cooking to keep variety and taste in Jim's diet. Mealtime is much more pleasurable now for Jim, and the foods are easier for him to swallow.

Grooming

A stroke can affect your self-image. You may not feel like a "whole" person. Or you may have neglect on one side of your body and not remember to take care of it. But good grooming, among other things, can help raise your spirits and make you feel more like yourself. Hygiene aside, good grooming is important to maintain after a stroke because it is good for self-esteem.

Anyone who has had a stroke should be encouraged to get out of pajamas and back into regular daywear as soon as possible. Pajamas and bed clothes tend to reinforce the self-image that you are "ill."

Especially if you are hemiplegic, however, some kinds of dressing will be harder than other kinds, so some adjustments in terms of style may be a good idea. Experiment with clothing and see what you like. Pullovers, which can be disorienting because they go on over the head, can be hard to put on. Tight-fitting clothing is not recommended, either.

Conventional clothing is often difficult for some stroke survivors to manage. Such clothing also may feel too restrictive. "Easy on/ easy off" clothing presents a useful alternative to conventional dressing. The Appendix has a partial list of mail-order sources for easy on/easy off clothing (see pages 293–294). These companies offer clothes for both men and women, and include everything from dresses, pants, and shirts to undergarments and shoes.

Check with members of stroke clubs or support groups in your area for the names of local shops that may carry easy on/easy off clothing as well.

Some movements will take a good deal of practice to master. Buttoning, tying laces, and snapping snaps can all be hard at first. You may want to practice these steps with the pants, shoes, shirt, or blouse in your lap. Try using a footstool when you are putting on shoes and socks. Remember to give the process time. And consult with your occupational therapist for additional ideas.

Dressing and Undressing

Undressing is a little easier to master, so it might make sense to start with that job first. When taking off shirts or pants, pull out the stronger limb first, and follow with the weaker one.

GROOMING AND SKIN CARE
IF YOU'VE HAD A STROKE

Your stroke may affect your image of yourself. Keeping your body clean and well groomed will help you feel more attractive. In fact, taking extra care of yourself will help you feel more complete. Wearing pajamas or a hospital gown in the daytime may make you think of yourself as a "sick" person, so wear your regular street clothes when you get home. Dressing up will help your self-image; you'll start thinking of yourself as "well" again.

Here are some other grooming tips:

• If you wore jewelry or makeup before your stroke, continue to do so.

• Use an electric shaver if you have to shave with one hand.

• Brush your teeth or dentures once or twice a day. This may even make your food taste better.

• If you can't shower, shampoo your hair by bending your head over a basin held on your lap and having someone pour water on your head from a pitcher. Comb or set your hair in a special way if doing so makes you feel more attractive.

• You may need to use an underarm deodorant now, especially on your weaker side, even if you didn't have to before.

• Keep your body clean and dry to prevent damage to your skin and to protect it from cuts. If your skin gets dry, irritated, or sore, give it special treatment immediately with a cream or lotion.

• People who clench their fists after a stroke should keep their fingernails short and smooth so they won't cut themselves. If you have this problem, soaking your hands daily will help keep them clean.

• Cut and file your toenails straight across after soaking them in warm water. Clean and dry the area between your toes carefully, and wear clean socks or stockings every day. If you're diabetic, consult your nurse about special foot care, and don't cut your own toenails!

• Clean your genital area and the area between your buttocks daily. Clean these areas more often if you have diarrhea or have trouble controlling your urine or stool. You may find cleaning yourself is easier when you're lying down.

When you're getting dressed, start by clothing your affected side first, using the unaffected side. Then dress the unaffected side. Steps to follow might go like this:

1. Lay out all the clothes you'll need in order. Clothes you'll need first should go on the top of the pile.
2. Put the weaker limb in the sleeve or leg of the clothing article first. Then arrange the clothing a bit before putting the stronger limb, or the head, through the appropriate openings.
3. Use your body weight to arrange the clothing around yourself.
4. Sit, rather than lie down, to dress yourself.

Some people have trouble dressing themselves after a stroke, not because of a physical disability, but because of a cognitive one. This is called **dressing apraxia.** These people have a spatial dysfunction. They can see what needs to be done, but they lack the sense of spatial perspective to do it correctly. They may try to button a shirt, but button it in the wrong order. Or they may try to apply lipstick, but miss their lips in the process.

If you have this problem, it helps if the people around you can give you clear instructions and hints to simplify the task. Keep your garments simple to reduce potential confusion. Learn how to position your clothes first. You might do this by practicing with a family member while holding the clothing in your lap. Look for the labels—they can help remind you which is the "right" side and which is the "wrong" side of the garment.

_____

"I'm worried about your mother," Norman told his daughter. "Since coming home from the hospital, she's just been lounging around in the house. She doesn't seem to want to get dressed or anything. And you know your mother—she's always been a pretty natty dresser."

It was true. Patricia had closets full of stylish clothes that she hadn't even looked at since her stroke. Her daughter Maria decided to find out what was wrong.

"I want to wear those clothes, dear, it's just that they're

too hard to put on and take off, I'm afraid," Patricia told Maria later that day. "Too many buttons and zippers and bows and whatnot. And anyway, those clothes are all pretty formal. I'm in more of an informal, comfortable mode these days. But I just don't know where to look for clothes like that."

Maria called a few places and learned that several of the largest national department store chains, as well as a number of smaller specialty stores, offered clothes that were specifically designed to be easy to put on and take off. She ordered their catalogs and had a wonderful time looking through them with her mother, who ordered several outfits.

Until they came, Maria worked with her mother to help her learn how to dress and undress herself, despite the paralysis of her left arm. Patricia found it was easier to dress her weaker side first and undress it last. She found snaps easier to work than buttons, and loop-and-pile-type closures the easiest of all. Zippers turned out to be easy enough to work if she could zip them from the front, and especially if she put a pom-pom or some other decorative bob on the end to hold onto as she pulled it up.

When the new clothes arrived, Patricia was delighted. She was able to dress herself again, and it was fun to have a few new outfits. Getting dressed up again gave her the self-esteem boost she needed. Soon she and Maria began going on weekly outings together. Sometimes they went to the cosmetics counters and sometimes the hairdresser. Sometimes they just went to the park.

Norman was pleased with Patricia's renewed interest in her activities. He was also glad he didn't have to go shopping. He gladly stayed home—and made the shoppers dinner when they returned.

Bathing

The bathroom is a fairly dangerous place for anyone, but especially so for those with disabilities. You may need a new bathing routine after you've had a stroke. The following tips may make bathing safer and easier. Refer also to the section on bathroom adaptations and transfers (pages 178–182 and 188–195).

- Set up everything before you begin to bathe. Put your soap, washcloth, towels, etc., all together.
- Test the water before getting into the tub, or ask someone else to test it for you. The water should not be too hot.
- Hand-held shower heads and long-handled brushes, loofahs, or terry-cloth mittens can make bathing easier.
- Until you are fully recovered, it isn't wise to shower or bathe without someone in attendance. Even then, it's a good idea to keep a bell handy. You can use it to call for help if needed.
- After you get out of the tub or shower, dry off completely. Rub yourself with lotion to prevent chapping.

Sexuality

If you're like most people, your sexual interest will remain the same after a stroke as it was before. But a stroke can cause physical and emotional changes where sexuality is concerned, depending on which part of the brain has been affected. Medications may affect sex, too. Men may have difficulty getting an erection or ejaculating. Women may have less feeling in the vagina or less lubrication.

Men and women who have had a stroke may feel inhibited or embarrassed by their bodies, have low self-esteem because of their stroke, or neglect sex because they are too tired. This can create feelings of tension and anxiety, and it can lead to conflicts between partners.

Returning to a satisfying sex life may require some changes. Both partners need to work to accommodate changes in body awareness, speech loss, and other deficits. But it certainly can be done. These suggestions may help you start to think about what kinds of changes might be useful:

- Stay as attractive as you can, through good grooming and personal hygiene.

MAKING DRESSING EASIER

These items can help make dressing with a disability easier.

• Rings or strings on zipper pulls

• Closures you can press together (loop-and-pile-type fasteners)

• Elastic waistbands

• Snaps and grippers

• Button hooks

• Elastic shoelaces or other simple shoe closures

• Sock/stocking spreaders (these can be made from old X-ray film)

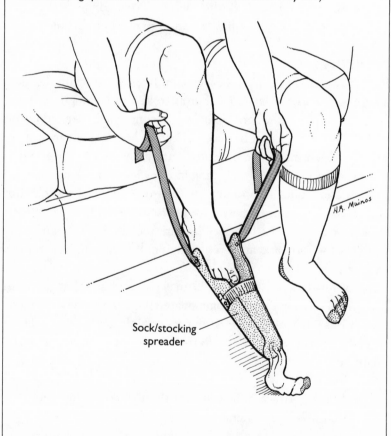

Sock/stocking spreader

- Talk openly with your partner about different needs and other changes that the stroke may have prompted.
- Plan in advance for sex, if possible. Choose times when both of you will be rested. Set aside plenty of time, with no interruptions.
- Try relaxing together before you begin. Soak in a bath, listen to music, or have a massage, for example.
- Be realistic. Old positions may not make sense. Find comfortable positions that support the weaker side and that conserve energy.
- A water-soluble, sterile lubricant may make penetration easier. Avoid petroleum jelly—it doesn't dissolve in water, and it may cause vaginal infection.
- Consider alternatives. Hugging, kissing, caressing, massaging, and touching can all be satisfying ways to show love and affection.

Not everyone develops problems with sexuality as the result of a stroke. Those who do, however, may wish to talk with their doctor, a qualified counselor, or a sex therapist about their problems.

Since her stroke, Joan hadn't felt very attractive. One side of her body drooped, which hurt her pride. Often she felt too tired to make herself up as she used to do. Because of her physical deficits, she wasn't sure she could resume her sexual relationship with her husband. And because of the way she felt about herself, she wasn't even sure he wanted to.

These feelings chased themselves around in Joan's mind for several weeks. Her husband could tell something was wrong, but Joan had been so withdrawn lately he didn't dare ask what it was. Finally, Joan decided just to say what was on her mind.

"Phil, I just don't feel very attractive right now. I so want to be close to you, but I'm afraid you won't want to be close to me, now that I've had this stroke. Is there anything I can do?"

Phil was taken utterly by surprise. He had thought all this

time that his wife simply didn't feel well enough for sex yet. He hastened to assure her that he was as in love with her as he had always been. He'd just thought she looked tired and might not appreciate resuming sex regularly.

They wound up having a long talk, voicing all of their worries and laying them to rest, one by one.

Finally, they decided to enjoy a "date" at home together the next evening. Joan chose the music to play softly on the stereo. Phil arranged to have dinner delivered from their favorite restaurant. They cleaned up the house together that morning and took it easy in the afternoon, so they wouldn't be tired that evening. Phil built a fire and Joan arranged some flowers in a vase on the table. At 5:30, they turned down the telephone so they couldn't be interrupted.

They dressed in separate bathrooms and took special pains to look their best. Promptly at six, Phil appeared and asked quite charmingly if Joan would care to join him for dinner. And just as charmingly, she said she would be delighted.

After a leisurely meal in the dining room, the couple retired to the living room and settled themselves on the old couch before the fireplace. They cuddled and caressed and talked until late, quite content with one another. The date had been a success, and their loving resumed quite naturally from there.

Getting Out and About

Independence and mobility are major issues for the person who is disabled. For most people in our society, the ability to get around town in a car is critical for doing shopping, getting to the doctor or to a place of worship, or maintaining social activities. If you don't have transportation, your sense of isolation can become great. It's well worth giving some time and consideration to transportation needs from the start.

Madeline had always been a busy person, on lots of commit-tees, with lots of responsibilities, and with lots of places she just liked to go. Now she was terribly frustrated. A stroke had left her with a visual deficit on the left side of her field of vision. Now she wasn't allowed to drive to any of her engagements. Not wanting to burden anyone else with her problems, Mad-eline simply stayed home instead of asking friends for rides. She withdrew a little bit.

With Madeline, withdrawing even a little bit was noticeable, however. Her friends all wondered why she had been missing meetings and lunches with them. Eleanor was elected to call and find out.

"It's such a pain, Eleanor," Madeline complained. "You just can't imagine. I loathe asking people for rides places. But I can't drive myself. It's not allowed, because of my stroke.

"Herb works all day, but he's offered to run errands for me at lunch, and of course evenings and weekends. I just haven't gotten used to it yet. I'll figure something out."

Eleanor was annoyed. "Why didn't you ask us in the first place, Madeline? Would you resent it if we called you for a ride? After all, we used to take turns shuttling our kids around to swim meets and baseball games and whatnot. We can cer-tainly take turns getting you to our meetings, lunches, and what have you. We want you there, so of course we don't mind giving you a ride. Please don't give it another thought."

Madeline accepted Eleanor's offer with grace. She really had missed her friends and involvements. Maybe Eleanor was right. She decided to take the initiative and see what some of her other options were. She got off the phone with Eleanor and then rang up the rapid transit office in her city to get a copy of the bus schedules and fares.

Two weeks later, Eleanor ran into Madeline at the mall. Madeline looked wonderful. The two women decided to have tea together. Madeline announced that she had taken the bus to the mall that morning. She had been getting reacquainted with the stores there. "You know, I feel so much better know-ing I can get around by myself again," Madeline said. "Herb and my son Nick have been great. They'll drive me anyplace I want to go, and that comes in handy a lot. But sometimes a woman just has to go her own way, you know?"

Eleanor said she certainly understood that. When they had finished their tea, Eleanor asked if she could drop Madeline anywhere. "That depends on where you're going," Madeline said waggishly.

"How about home? I'm pooped," Eleanor said. "Your house is on my way, you know."

"Then, yes, I'd appreciate that very much, Eleanor," Madeline said immediately. "Thank you for offering." The two women paid for their tea and moved off into the mall crowd.

Some people who have had a stroke worry that they will not be able to drive anymore. In fact, some kinds of disabilities do make driving a very dangerous activity. Some stroke survivors have severe visual impairments. Others may have cognitive disabilities that make them poor judges of their environment. These people should not drive, for their own safety as well as others'. For many of them, public transportation can fill in the gap. In some cases, however, people who have had strokes may be able to drive again.

The first thing to do if you are considering driving again after your stroke is to ask your doctor about the possibility. Do not assume that you are OK and ready to take the wheel.

If your doctor thinks you might be able to drive again, the next step is to call the Department of Motor Vehicles in your area. Ask to speak with someone in the Office of Driver Safety. Identify yourself, tell the officer that you have had a stroke, and describe any deficits you may have. Ask about special requirements they may have for you. You may have to take a driving test and install special equipment in your car, for example.

Some areas have specialized businesses that will evaluate your driving if you have had a stroke. For a fee, which may be deductible under some insurance policies, they will test your vision, reaction speed, and driving. Usually the evaluation is made partly in a clinic and partly in a vehicle that they provide. If you pass, they will notify the Department of Motor Vehicles for you. You will need a valid license and a prescription from your doctor to be evaluated. If you are interested, ask about driver evaluation services at your local rehab center. If you need retraining, be sure you find a qualified instructor. Ask your rehabilitation center for a referral, or take a certified driver's education class.

Many parking lots reserve spaces close to the entrances of buildings for those who are disabled. These places are usually identified by the blue-and-white international wheelchair symbol. To use that parking, you'll need to submit a written disability statement from your doctor to your local police headquarters. The police will issue the permit. If you can drive, obtain a special license plate through your state's Department of Motor Vehicles.

If you can't drive a car yourself, or do not wish to drive, public transportation may be a good alternative for you. Many cities offer reduced-fare passes for older people or people who are disabled. Wheelchair lifts are available on more and more buses. In other cases, some cities will provide wheelchair-accessible vans for your trips around town. These vans may be available by appointment only, however, so you may have to plan trips a bit in advance. Some agencies may even provide you with an escort.

It may pay to use your creativity to find public transportation tailored to your needs and schedule. Some senior citizens' groups may have information on door-to-door service for those who are sixty years old or more. Local volunteer agencies may offer ride services. Check too with your State Department on Aging for special services that might help you.

After you have found a way to reach your destination, you may get there only to find that you can't get in because of physical barriers. If possible, try to call ahead to make sure that the building is accessible to you.

Some major cities publish access guides. These tell which public buildings, theaters, shopping centers, restaurants, and the like have handicap facilities.

Travel

Travel doesn't need to stop after a stroke. It may take a little extra preparation, however, to make sure everything goes as smoothly as possible. Most carriers, whether airplane, bus, or train, can accommodate the traveler with special needs. Here's how you can help them help you:

1. Plan ahead. Make your reservation well in advance.
2. Give complete information. At the time that you make your reservation, describe precisely the kinds of services you will need. If you have a wheelchair, say whether you want to transport your own chair or use their equipment from station to station (if available). Let them know if your wheelchair is battery-operated or not. Identify any other special equipment or needs you may have. If you need a low-fat or low-sodium meal, for example, they may be able to provide it with advance notice.
3. Allow extra time at check-in. Always allow plenty of time to check in and get settled before plane flights and train or bus trips. Ask how much time they suggest when you make your reservation.

Before starting your trip, be sure to find out what kind of access and special services are available at the places you will be visiting. Major hotel chains sometimes list in their directories the special services they offer at individual hotels. Call ahead to confirm. Never assume special services will be provided anywhere. Special assistance is available at most train stations—but not all of them.

Once your trip has begun, a few other tips can help make the experience more pleasant:

- Wear loose, casual clothing.
- Be sure to carry identification with you. Include your complete name and address.
- Carry a list of emergency contact numbers with you. Include the names and phone numbers of a relative or close friend, your doctor, your insurance carrier, information on drug allergies, etc.
- Carry a list of your medications, along with their dosages and consumption schedules.

- Keep with you any medicines you might need in an emergency.

Travelers with disabilities may be interested in joining the Society for the Advancement of Travel for the Handicapped. All members receive a newsletter and some publications. Some areas hold chapter meetings. For more information, write to them at the address given in the Appendix (see page 293).

Coping with Sensory and Perceptual Problems —Tips for the Person Who Is Disabled

A stroke can affect your ability to see, hear, touch, move about, and think. A disability in any of these areas might cause a sensory or perceptual problem. Sometimes people with these problems aren't aware that they have them. This puts them at greater risk of accidental injury around the home. Occupational therapists have training programs that emphasize activities performed on a repetitive and sequential basis. This training is often useful in coping with perceptual deficits. If you have such deficits, here are some general safety ideas that may help you avoid accidents. Your occupational therapist may have further suggestions as well.

1. Keep your home neat and free of hazards.
2. Follow a daily routine.
3. Eliminate background distractions while you're doing a difficult task. You need to be able to concentrate your thoughts on the task at hand.
4. Work slowly. This, too, helps you focus on the steps involved in the task.
5. Ask for help. If needed, a caregiver or family member should be ready, willing, and able to help out.

Sensory Problems

If you have sensory impairment, your feelings of pain, temperature, and pressure can be compromised. This can present an enormous safety hazard to you. Even such familiar things as hot water, sharp knives, and electrical appliances can be dangerous if you're not able to tell if you've been injured or not. If you have any sensory impairment, be extra careful in your actions everywhere, but especially in the kitchen and bath. (Some safety ideas for the kitchen and bath are given in previous sections.)

Visual Problems

Visual problems of various types are fairly common among stroke survivors. Some people lose half of their visual field in one eye. This condition is called **hemianopia.** (If both eyes are equally affected, the condition is called **homonymous hemianopia.**) It can be a safety risk, because you're more likely to bump into things, like doorways, on your blind side. It can also make some tasks, such as reading or dressing, initially harder to do. Driving with this condition can be extremely dangerous. Be sure to check with your doctor before attempting to drive. Fortunately, this condition usually improves in the weeks following the stroke.

A person with either condition is taught to compensate for the blind half of his visual field by turning his head frequently and scanning. If either condition is accompanied by neglect, however, rehabilitation becomes harder. Family and friends can help by reminding the person with hemianopia to pay active attention to his impaired side.

Judging distance accurately can also be compromised by a stroke. In this case, your perception of space is affected. As the warning on the rearview mirror of a car says, "Objects are actually closer than they appear." Or they may appear closer. This can cause you to bump into things, misjudge steps, or overreach or underreach for objects. It helps consciously to think about where the objects are —near, far, or in the middle distance—before acting. Managing stairs can obviously be dangerous unless you take great care. Use the handrail and feel for the height of the step before shifting your weight to that leg. Someone should help support your weaker side as well.

It may also be hard to distinguish between objects that are in a pile or that are the same color. This problem often comes up where laundry is concerned, when socks are all piled together in a drawer, or when buttons are the same color as the shirts they are attached to. The following ideas may help if you have this problem. You can probably think of even more ways to make things work better for you.

1. As recommended for anyone with sensory or perceptual problems, be sure to keep your home neat and tidy.
2. Keep items you use often within easy reach. Keep that area well organized.
3. Sort clothing into stacks that make it easy to get the items you need.
4. If dressing is a problem, become oriented to each garment by locating the neck opening first, then a sleeve or leg, etc.
5. Ask someone to sew buttons on your clothing in contrasting colors. Use contrasting colors for dishes and placemats, pillows and sheets, handles and drawers.

Hearing Problems

Usually strokes don't cause a hearing loss, although they can interfere with the brain's ability to interpret what is heard. It's easy enough to determine the difference with a hearing test. If you wore a hearing aid before the stroke, you'll need one afterward as well. If you're buying a hearing aid for the first time, check the store's return policy. You may be able to rent or borrow one before buying it. That way you may return it if it is uncomfortable or isn't right for you in any other way.

Cognitive Problems

If you've had a stroke in the frontal lobes of the brain, you may have memory lapses or problems planning and following through on a task, among other things. These kinds of disabilities are frustrating and discouraging and often very alarming to your loved ones. Although precise strategies for relearning a task vary according to the deficit, some basic approaches apply for most cases.

1. Use simple, step-by-step directions.
2. Be patient; practice the task many times.
3. Slow down and take all the time you need. There is no hurry, and it may be safer to go more slowly.
4. Learn new ways to do things instead of trying to do everything the way you did it before. Occupational therapy specialists can be of particular help here.

Living with a Disability: Tips for the Family

Physical and behavioral changes can be difficult not only for the person who has had a stroke but also for her loved ones. They may become impatient with the stroke survivor's slow progress with walking or her messiness at the table. They may be puzzled by behavioral changes that seem to have no physical cause—sudden bouts of crying, harsh cursing, or a new indifference to her surroundings. These may only become apparent when the stroke survivor gets home. In this section, we'll look at some ways in which caregivers, family, and friends might learn to live with another's disability in some major areas.

Neglect

Neglect has been called a "disorder of attention." A person with neglect has a number of sensory deficits on the stroke-involved side of the body. A person with neglect ignores or is indifferent to everything on that side. This disorder is more common among those with right-brain damage (and left hemiplegia) than vice versa.

The severity of neglect varies from one person to the next. For some, the effects can be severe; for others, only mild. Neglect comes in several forms, called **extinction, anosognosia,** and **somatognosia.** People with extinction ignore stimulation on their affected side. Those with anosognosia might show anything from an unconcern for their paralysis, to a denial of their paralysis, to an outright denial that the affected limb or limbs are their own. Anosognosia is a particularly severe form of neglect to treat because of the person's indifference to his disability. A person with somatognosia has a hard time perceiving how the impaired side of his body relates to everything else around him. He may confuse another person's limbs for his own, for example.

Neglect affects not only the way the person perceives sensations on the impaired side of the body but also the way he perceives any input coming from that side. Often there is a visual component to neglect. The person ignores food on one side of his plate, words on one side of a page, even visitors who face him from the impaired side of his body.

Common Problems
Neglect can present a variety of problems that caregivers should look out for.

Accidents. Injuries can be a problem for a person with neglect. If he is paralyzed, his indifference to or denial of his affected limb can mean that he tries to walk—only to fall down. In addition, because he doesn't recognize his affected side, he won't try to protect himself from potential injury to it.

Isolation. A stroke survivor with neglect selectively ignores everything on one side of his body. Thus he can become extremely isolated if the unimpaired side isn't stimulated. He needs visual input, conversation, etc., throughout the course of the day. The person with neglect should not be seated with his unimpaired side next to a wall and then left alone, for example. Position his unaffected side to where the action is, unless you are specifically working with the affected side. After dark, a night-light or soft music from a radio that is placed on the unimpaired side may be comforting.

Many stroke survivors are older and may already have some visual or hearing impairments that are isolating—neglect can only worsen those feelings. In a person with neglect, it is a good idea to try to involve the neglected side in daily activity drills. We'll discuss that shortly.

Confusion. Moving about or traveling can become confusing to a person with neglect, because what he notices going in one direction is not the same as what he sees on the return trip. It helps if the caregiver points out landmarks on either side along the way and refers frequently to the destination. This holds true whether the caregiver accompanies the stroke survivor just down the hall or all the way to Aunt Mary's house in the next county.

Resistance to Rehabilitation. Because they can't recognize that they have a problem on the affected side, people with neglect are often indifferent to rehabilitation efforts that could be very helpful. The degree of their resistance varies with the degree of their neglect.

What to Do to Help

Occupational and speech therapy may be the best way to help the stroke survivor with neglect learn some tasks. But there is a lot that caregivers, friends, and family can do to help, too. The idea is to get the person to begin to recognize his impaired side and to develop other cues to compensate for this deficit. The way to do that is to work with the impaired side in daily activities with the person and refer to it often in conversations with him. As mentioned earlier, if you are working with the person, you might position him so that his unimpaired side is turned away from the action—the opposite of what you would normally do. This helps him concentrate on you and his neglected side better.

Depending on the extent of the neglect, many stroke survivors can learn over time to compensate for this deficit and acknowledge their neglected side. Here are some ways to help.

- Give the person plenty of feedback about the neglected side. Refer to it in conversation. For example, ask the person to point out body parts he neglects. Identify something on his neglected side and ask him to point it out to you. This helps him relearn recognition of that side.
- Involve that side physically. Touch, move, and look at the limbs on the affected side and have the person

do so, too. Put the limbs on that side in a natural position as you work with your loved one.

- Encourage the person's attention to the neglected side. Attach a bright ribbon, watch, or bell to that wrist and encourage him to pay attention to it. Try putting a bright strip of tape or a bright shoelace on the shoe of the affected foot. A scented lotion rubbed only on the affected arm might also help.

- Work from the neglected side. This encourages the person to scan his environment for input and not rely on his unimpaired side alone for information. Sit on the affected side when working with the person. Visitors might approach the person from his neglected side while calling his name (and some might sit on that side, too). At the dinner table, the person might receive food from his non-neglected side, but be asked to pass it across to his neglected side.

  It may be a good idea to divide bedside articles between the person's impaired and unimpaired sides, if he is confined to bed. The most necessary articles should remain on the person's unaffected side so he can get to them quickly and easily if he is alone. But those that are less necessary might go on the other table. This may entice the person to "hunt" for them. (The idea here is not to make the person feel persecuted, of course, but to encourage him to explore the full range of his environment.)

- Don't nag. Simply nagging the person to turn his head and acknowledge something on his neglected side doesn't work. Instead, give cues and gently draw the person's attention to his neglected side. You might mention a ring on his finger while holding that hand, for example. And although problems of neglect can be very frustrating for everyone, try to maintain a pleasant tone of voice and be encouraging. A person with neglect needs your support.

- Alter the environment. If neglect is so severe as to be disabling, or if it persists, it may be wise to simply acknowledge the condition and alter the stroke survivor's environment. A favorite chair in the living room and the contents of drawers, for example, might all be rearranged to favor the person's non-neglected side. Doing so maximizes his independence and performance.

Aphasia

Aphasia is a general term that describes a variety of communication deficits. (See pages 98–99 for a complete discussion of aphasia.) An aphasia can affect a person's ability to express himself to others through spoken or written language. It can also affect his ability to comprehend the spoken or written language of others. The person's ability to use or interpret body language may also be affected. Strokes may make the physical articulation of speech difficult for the stroke survivor. The different types of aphasia are discussed in greater detail in Chapter Three (see pages 98–99) and reviewed briefly below. The severity of aphasia differs from one person to the next. Generally, the more severe the stroke, the worse the resulting aphasia. Sometimes aphasias disappear or become much less noticeable with time.

In Wernicke's aphasia, the stroke survivor is unable to understand language. The goal when working with such a person is to help him recognize that he has a language problem and to help him improve the quality of his speech. To do this, it's a good idea to provide examples of correct speech, rather than to correct the person endlessly. Reading aloud slowly may be a useful drill. It's also a good idea to work on nonverbal means of communication between the person and others. Pantomime and facial expressions could be part of this.

The person with Wernicke's aphasia may find spoken language scrambled and confusing. Try to keep things as simple for him as possible. It might be a good idea to work with this person in a quiet room. Avoid extraneous noise or visual clutter that might distract him.

In Broca's aphasia, the person has difficulty expressing himself. The goal in helping someone with this condition is to get the person to use words again in a consistent way. Repetitive language drills help in this regard. They may involve sentence completion, yes or no responses to questions, and object identification. Singing sometimes helps the person control his speech, so he may benefit by singing sentences, words, or phrases.

Not every hospital has speech and language specialists available. The organizations listed in the Appendix can provide information on aphasia (see pages 290–293). They can also refer stroke survivors to qualified specialists in their area.

Dealing with a person with aphasia can be a confusing experience for his family, because his problems seem to be so selective. He may not speak, yet seem to understand what is said to him. Or he may talk a lot—without making any sense. How to communicate in the face of a language deficit of any kind can be a perplexing and frustrating proposition. But it can be done. Remember that speaking and writing are just two of the many ways humans communicate with each other. We also use body language, pantomime, music, and other methods to get our points across. The key to learning to communicate with an aphasic person is to stay flexible in your notions of what "communication" is. The following tips may help.

- Remember that the person with aphasia hasn't necessarily lost his ability to think clearly. Even if he doesn't speak or is hard to understand, he probably understands more than he can express, so don't say anything in front of him that you don't want him to hear. And don't freeze him out of family decision making. Be sure to include him, especially if the issues under discussion concern him directly.
- Prepare the area for conversation. Quiet, calm surroundings are less distracting for someone with aphasia. Try to minimize distractions in the room around you so that the person has an easier time concentrating on communication.
- Speak directly to the person. Position yourself within his line of vision, especially if he has hemianopia (partial blindness) or other vision problems. It may help him understand more if he can watch your lips move and gauge your facial expression, body movements, and the like.

- Simplify your communication. Try not to overload your speech with complex ideas. Speak in short, precise sentences. Use familiar words. Pause between sentences.
- Don't assume the person has a hearing problem. It may seem as though someone with a receptive aphasia doesn't hear you. Usually, however, he hears fine—the problem is he doesn't understand what he hears. If you have doubts, a hearing test can resolve the question.

  Don't shout while speaking to him. Although it may seem that shouting works, it probably isn't because the person hears you better. Shouting takes energy, and most of us shout in very short bursts, using simple language to get our point across. It's that concision that the person may be responding to and understanding—not the loudness. When talking to someone with aphasia, do speak slowly and use single words or short sentences to communicate—but don't yell.
- Give the aphasic adequate time to respond. It may take thirty seconds or more for him to digest what you have said and then reply. Be patient.
- Don't condescend. A person with aphasia tends to understand shorter sentences and phrases better than longer, more complex ones. Thus it can be tempting to use a "special voice" when talking with him. This is never necessary, and understandably it may anger some people or hurt their feelings. Speak to a person with aphasia in the same tone as you would to any other adult. And try to pick subjects to talk about that reflect his interests.
- Enrich the communication experience. Depending on the sort of aphasia the person has, it may be a good idea to use pictures, photos, gestures, and sounds to supplement your efforts to communicate with him. If the stroke has not affected his ability to read, you might try using written materials, too.
- Be patient and encouraging. It's tiring and frustrating not to be understood or not to understand others. It's

very likely that the person will frequently become angry during the slow process of relearning communication skills. Don't take it personally. Instead, try to convey that you understand why he is angry. If possible, try to identify any specific sources of his frustration and take care of them.

It's also important that you don't betray your own frustrations or raise your voice when trying to communicate. Consider taking a short break if either you or the person is too frustrated to continue cheerfully.

Praise progress, but do so in a genuine way. Empty praise just isn't helpful, and it can become annoying.

• Be honest if you haven't understood. It's perfectly okay to tell the person you haven't understood him, as long as you avoid doing so in a critical way. Encourage him to try again.

Gestures, pointing, writing, or using a word board are other ways in which someone with aphasia might be able to communicate effectively with others. A speech specialist can determine which alternative may be most effective.

• Go with what works. If the person seems to use a made-up word consistently for one meaning, don't insist that he use the "correct" word instead. If you can both understand, there isn't a problem.

"Quality Control" Problems

After a stroke, some people may have difficulty with "social judgment," or the ability to know what to do, when. Formerly neat people may become sloppy and inattentive about their grooming. Formerly quiet people may burst out with vulgar language at inappropriate times, for no apparent reason. These problems, and others like them, are usually first picked up on by those who are closest to the person who has had a stroke. The changes they notice are often annoying. They can also be confusing, because often the person's other mental processes remain sharp. These problems are easy to mistake for emotional or psychological problems. Although such problems may be a factor, it's important that professionals first try to sort out any stroke deficits that may be behind the behavior.

COMMUNICATING WITH SOMEONE WHO HAS APHASIA

A person with aphasia is one who has partially or completely lost the ability to speak or to understand speech. The inability to communicate with her can be a painful and frustrating experience. The following changes in the way we communicate may help.

Simplify. Present one idea at a time. Use short sentences with simple words. Speak slowly but naturally.

Be clear. Be sure that you have the aphasic person's attention before you begin to speak. Use gestures. Repeat or reword the idea until the person understands. Confusion is likely to increase with noise and activity.

Allow time. Be patient, accepting the person's speech attempts, and don't hurry her.

Guess. Try to find out the subject of the person's concern. You may do this by asking specific questions such as, "Is it about the hospital?"

Confirm. Make statements about what you think she means, to be sure that you understand. Find out if the person can say "Yes" or "No." If the aphasic person says "Yes" to a question and you are not sure if the question was understood, ask the opposite. If the person again answers "Yes," then you are not communicating.

Be honest. Say, "I'm sorry, I don't understand you," when necessary. Then reassure the person and try again.

Respect. The aphasic person is often aware of what is happening even though her language function is impaired. Include her in conversation.

Quality control problems can result from memory deficits, visual deficits, and even minor speech deficits.

People with aphasia often feel isolated because they can't talk and express themselves. They may act out their feelings of anxiety instead. Sulking, lack of cooperation, mood swings, or a sudden refusal to participate in therapy may be signs of this.

Talk over any worries or questions you have about this kind of problem with your doctor. The more you know, the better you can adjust. Information and reminders can help people with social difficulties recognize the problem and help them modify their behavior over time. Have patience and give them your support and encouragement. Don't withdraw because you disapprove of the behavior, because often the person can't help it. Social exclusion will only reinforce his discouragement. Above all, he needs to be reassured that he is still accepted by family and friends.

Coping with Stroke —A Psychological Adjustment for the Stroke Survivor and the Family

Stroke is undoubtedly one of the most traumatic and stressful events that can befall a person. At the hospital, much emphasis is placed on making the fullest physical recovery possible. Yet learning to adjust psychologically to the changes stroke has introduced into the stroke survivor's life can be equally important for a truly satisfactory recovery. Coping deserves its own place in the recovery process.

Chen's family was very worried about him. Ever since his severe stroke the month before, he had been acting very strange. He had aphasia and couldn't understand what people tried to tell him. He seemed to have given up on trying to communicate. In fact, he just sort of shut down. He cried frequently, too, which wasn't at all like him.

Elaine, Chen's wife, and their grown sons knew this behavior was unusual and that it probably required professional help. First they discussed Chen's aphasia with his speech therapy specialist. They wanted to see if there was anything they could do to lessen Chen's frustration.

"Just keep trying," Cheryl told them. "If talking doesn't seem to work, try pantomiming. Try using pictures to communicate. Be positive around him, too," she said, "but be yourselves. Reassure him and encourage him to stay relaxed. He's been through a big change, and it's going to take time for everyone to adjust."

Still, despite their efforts, Chen seemed to withdraw more and more. Now he was refusing to participate in his physical therapy exercises, too. The family spoke with Chen's physician next.

"I wanted to see if we could shake this without resorting to medications, but if Chen isn't participating in his physical therapy, that could just complicate his health down the road," Dr. Michaelson said thoughtfully. "We'll try this for a little while and see if it helps. I think if we can just get him through this, he'll be OK."

Dr. Michaelson put Chen on antidepressant medication and monitored him carefully. The family noticed that Chen's mood seemed to improve. He began to respond again to their efforts at communication. His speech and physical therapy began to show more progress, too.

The family was greatly relieved. Now they felt they were back on track. But they knew they had a lot to learn about stroke and depression. Chen's illness, it was clear, had affected them, too. With Chen's agreement, the whole family joined a stroke support group. Every week they got together with other families that were experiencing the same things they were. It felt good to have a place where they could get their anger, fears, and confusion off their chests. The best part was being with other people who understood what they were going through.

***

Emotional distress is common after stroke. Stroke survivors may feel frustration, anxiety, or even depression. These feelings may go unreported by the person who has had the stroke or by his family members. Left without expression, these feelings can grow. They can then hamper rehabilitation and adjustment efforts and even create new problems.

Coping is a process that varies among individuals. It comprises three basic stages:

1. Loss. You may have experienced losses as a result of your stroke. You may have lost the use of an arm or

a leg, the ability to speak, the ability to read, general competence, pride, or a positive body image or self-image. The stage of loss reflects sadness at the awareness that your life has changed.

2. Appraisal. In this stage, you begin to examine what the stroke means for you. Sometimes a stroke deficit can prevent you from appraising your situation accurately.

3. Rebuilding. In this stage, you start to work on re-learning skills and making peace with any remaining disability.

The process of coping is enhanced by information and action. It helps both those who have had strokes and their families to get as much accurate and reassuring information about the stroke as possible. This activity helps everybody assimilate a very upsetting and foreign event into their lives so they can deal with it. Uncertainty is very stressful, and it makes coping difficult because it prevents people from making plans. The act of planning for the future is itself a coping mechanism.

Planning helps people feel they have some control over, or can accurately anticipate, their future. Working toward rehabilitation goals might be one good coping mechanism. Knowing the likelihood of a second stroke and working on goals to reduce those odds is another. These activities relieve stress, too.

Helping the Stroke Survivor Cope

Psychological adjustment after stroke is affected by a number of variables. If you were optimistic and hopeful before your stroke, you are more likely to cope well than someone who was originally more negative. (That person probably will require more reassurance.) A serious medical condition in addition to the stroke adds more stress, and it may affect your ability to cope well. Financial worry can add to the burden of stress. The quality of the home environment also can affect how well you cope with a traumatic event such as stroke.

If you or someone you know isn't coping well with stroke, remember that help is available. The American Heart Association's Stroke Connection can refer you to people who can help (see page

290). Religion and prayer, a circle of friends, a support group, and the resumption of favorite activities can all help bolster a person's sense of faith in the future.

Depression

Someone who isn't coping well with his stroke may show signs of withdrawal, depression, sleep disturbances, and indifference to therapy. He may be frustrated by new limitations imposed by the stroke, worried about recurrence, or feel isolated by his experience. As a caregiver, try to keep communication lines open. (If he is aphasic, you may need to find some creative alternative methods.) Allow the stroke survivor to express his fears. Encourage him to relax in relearning daily activities, and remind him that progress takes time. You as a caregiver or family member also need to be positive but realistic.

Some researchers have found that one-third to one-half of all stroke survivors become depressed at some point. Depression is a normal reaction to a traumatic event. Usually the depressed feelings are strongest soon after the stroke and subside with time.

If withdrawal or depression persists, however, discuss the matter with a doctor. Psychological, vocational, or peer counseling may help. (The doctor can refer you to the appropriate people.) If necessary, medication may be prescribed to treat the condition.

Moods and Mood Changes

Stroke survivors often have emotional problems. They may feel understandably sad or unaccountably cheerful. They may be sometimes irritable and unable to control their anger. They may seem withdrawn and indifferent or be impulsive. They may have unexplained mood changes.

Some stroke survivors experience outbursts of tears and sometimes laughter or anger. These expressions may match the person's feelings, but in an exaggerated way. Or they may be completely inappropriate. "Emotional lability" is a term used to describe such emotional experiences. Caregivers and family members need to understand that these incidents are a result of the stroke and are outside the stroke survivor's control. Being understanding about the incidents sometimes helps. In time, the stroke survivor may have spontaneous improvement and increased emotional control.

Other stroke survivors may seem apathetic: indifferent to everyday occurrences and unmoved by emotional events. In an extreme case, an apathetic survivor is unable to set goals, is unmotivated, and is unresponsive to urgent needs. She gets no pleasure from any activity. Apathy is usually a short-term problem. With understanding and encouragement from a caregiver, the stroke survivor usually regains her healthy emotional outlook.

These emotional events may seem very difficult to handle. Family members sometimes remark that the stroke survivor acts very different since the stroke. "She just isn't herself," is a phrase often used to describe the emotional aspect of a stroke survivor.

Remember that stroke represents a very large change in many lives. Stroke survivors and their families need time to adjust to these changes. Stroke support groups can be very helpful for both the stroke survivor and family members. Sometimes professional therapy is needed. A caregiver may feel that an emotional problem has gone on too long or has worsened. If so, he should talk to the stroke survivor's doctor about it. Don't hesitate to get professional care when necessary. Just remember, the outlook for most stroke survivors with emotional problems is excellent. Most learn to adjust to their conditions and enjoy life again.

Feeling Tired After a Stroke

Many stroke survivors feel fatigued after they come home from the hospital. Don't be alarmed if this happens to you. There are many reasons you may feel tired. You may have less energy than before. This can be because of a lack of sleep, proper exercise, or proper nutrition. You may have just as much energy as before the stroke, but just be using it in different ways. It often requires a great deal of effort to compensate for some physical deficits. Here are some ideas that may help you overcome these feelings of fatigue:

1. Tell your doctor how you feel. There may be some physical, emotional, or cognitive problem that needs further treatment.
2. Look at your energy level and that of the people around you. Structure your day in a way that works for all of you. Try to find a time of day that is best for you to do things together or just to talk.

3. Assign priorities to your activities. Decide what are the most important things for you to do in a day. Then do only those things on days when you feel low on energy. On high-energy days, add some activities with lower priority.

4. Use your energy wisely. Don't spend time and energy on things that you cannot change. Use aids that are appropriate for your level of ability. If walking without your cane makes you too tired one day, use it. If you find you do not need it the next day, try a walk without it. If you are planning to go a long distance, consider using a wheelchair instead of your cane.

5. If you feel tired from thinking, take a break from your activity and move around. Try swinging your arms, walking around, or having someone move you around a bit.

6. Develop the best communication skills you can. Find a clear, brief way to explain your limitations. Your rehabilitation team can help with this. A printed explanation you can give to others is sometimes very useful.

7. Don't hesitate to ask for help.

8. Try to find at least one way to release feelings of anger, sadness, fear, etc. This may be through breathing exercises, talking to someone, or using your body in some active way. Your doctor or other member of your rehabilitation team can help you find ways to do this.

9. Learn some ways to relax. Try a relaxing activity or even a nap.

10. Every day, do something you enjoy. Then show your enthusiasm for it.

11. Don't put yourself down.

12. Celebrate each of your successes, no matter how small.

The Importance of Activity

Once at home, you as a stroke survivor may have more time on your hands than you had in the hospital. Television and the radio simply aren't enough to fill that time. Hobbies, visits with friends, and household chores—as your strength and endurance allow—are all important activities and should be pursued. Some hobbies or activities that might appeal to you include reading, cards, crafts, indoor gardening, travel, and visiting others. There are even sports activities that can be done one-handed: horseshoes, table tennis, shuffleboard, darts, bowling, and fishing. As an interest develops, keep an eye out for adaptive equipment that could come in handy in this area. Card and book holders may be a good idea for many. Others may appreciate embroidery hoops that can clamp onto tables. These and many other hobby aids are widely available.

Even after you are well on the road to recovery, you may be separated from your familiar social environment. Physical deficits, changes in mental functioning, and emotional problems can all make social activities difficult. You may feel overwhelmed by a seemingly simple activity—talking on the phone, shopping, taking a walk, or going out to eat.

It is important for friends and relatives to help stroke survivors adjust to the changes in their lives. As a caregiver, be encouraging and helpful. Be sure to draw the stroke survivor into all home activities, including household planning sessions. Make a point of spending uninterrupted time with her. This attention is important to her self-esteem and shows more than anything that she is still very much respected and needed by the family.

Stroke Clubs and Stroke Support Groups

Stroke clubs and stroke support groups can be beneficial to a stroke survivor and his caregiver or family members. Some stroke clubs are social groups. Members share their experiences, swap useful information, and may share equipment or other resources. Others serve as support groups and are run by professional counselors. They provide formal group counseling and psychological support. These counselors are available for stroke survivors, their families, and caregivers. A stroke support group can be a helpful way of expressing and confronting frustrations, resentments, and anxieties in a directed way. Still others may be some combination of these two.

For information on stroke clubs and stroke support groups in your area, call your local American Heart Association, or the AHA's Stroke Connection (see page 290 for the address and phone number). They can also give you information on starting your own stroke club and can help you find specific information.

Helping the Family Cope

Family members and caregivers also experience a great deal of stress in the wake of a loved one's stroke. Their lives have changed after the stroke, too, and they need understanding and support. Information and action help them cope as well.

Bringing a stroke survivor home can be stressful for you as a caregiver or family member. Adequate preparation for this arrival helps. You need to have a realistic idea of what changes to expect in the household routine and in the stroke survivor himself. You need to know this before the stroke survivor returns home. If you are nervous about caring for the health and safety of the stroke survivor, you may wish to take a home nursing course through a local Red Cross agency. The skills you will learn are extremely useful, and learning them can help reduce your feelings of anxiety in this area.

You should continue to draw on community support resources, if they are available, to help care for the stroke survivor. One of these resources might be a caregiver's support group. As described above, this kind of group gives caregivers a place in which to blow off steam, vent frustrations, and share experiences with an empathic audience.

Perhaps most important, you need to allow yourself to take breaks from your role as a caregiver. You will need time to recharge your batteries and pursue your interests—in other words, to care for yourself. At home, divide care duties so one person isn't responsible for everything. The stroke survivor himself should begin to take responsibility for his own self-care and exercise, but he may need some help and extra time to do so, especially at first. Let friends help who have offered to. And don't be afraid to ask for their help, either. Sometimes friends who want to help don't, because they aren't sure what would be appreciated. Tell them!

You may also need to take longer breaks occasionally. Many resources available today can provide caregivers with time away from the home to run errands or relax. Your State Department on Aging can help you locate caregiver relief. The following are some of the kinds of agencies it may recommend.

Adult day care centers are usually aimed at seniors, and they provide a social setting and supervision for a few hours a day. They are meant for people who are fairly independent.

Respite care is available through some agencies. For a few hours or up to a few days, a nurse or therapist stays in the home while the regular caregiver takes a break. If a longer break is needed, some nursing-home facilities will accept patients for a one- or two-week stay.

Extended family and friends are often a trusted and willing resource for caregivers, as are fellow members of your church, synagogue, or other place of worship. Accept their offers of help if given, and don't hesitate to ask for help, either.

An exhausted, cranky caregiver doesn't do himself or anyone else much good. Take a rest when you need it. Get out and about for a short time during the day, or on a weekend, or for a longer period if necessary. Don't become isolated yourself because of your perceived responsibilities. You'll come back refreshed, with a more positive outlook. And that's good for everybody.

Community Resources

It can be difficult for people who have been independent all their lives to ask for help. Yet community service agencies exist to make life easier in some difficult areas for those who qualify. You may have paid for many of these services indirectly over the years, through your taxes or donations to organizations such as the United Way. Don't hesitate to investigate any services or programs that may help you (or your loved one) remain as independent as possible.

Sometimes finding the appropriate services that may be of help is a problem. Needs differ. Some stroke survivors need meals delivered; others just want information. A social worker or other specialist assigned to your stroke team at the hospital generally can help identify the right resources for you.

Keep in mind that getting a lot of different services may not be the best course of action. The goal is still to become as independent as possible. Ideally, you'll find a strategy that uses the fewest support services while providing you with maximum independence.

Community resources can be divided into social, vocational, financial, and legal services. Some programs are meant to provide temporary relief; others are for the long term.

Social Services

These include transportation needs and support groups. They also include alternative living arrangements, nursing care, and respite care. These have been discussed in Chapter Six, so we won't repeat that information here. But other social services, such as meals, homemaker help, and emergency alert services, may also be useful.

Meal programs help people who may not be able to shop for or prepare their own food. This includes those who have a deficit, are low-income, or are socially isolated. The programs may provide meals regularly or occasionally.

Senior centers, churches, synagogues, or public agencies may provide hot meals once a day in a group setting. Many of these programs are administered as part of a federal program called the Older Americans Act. Meals on Wheels, another federal program, provides hot meals in many areas. Volunteers deliver the meals directly to the home. This program is meant for shut-ins who are sixty years old or more. For more information on meal programs, contact your State Department on Aging office, a social worker, or your hospital.

Homemaker services are flexible services in which aides come to the home to help prepare meals and do house cleaning, laundry, and the like. This arrangement can be great for a person who wants to maintain his independence but can use an extra pair of hands around the house for some chores. Be sure to go through a reputable agency to hire anyone you don't know well. Home health care agencies, a social services department, senior citizen centers, and your State Department on Aging office may all be able to provide referrals in this area. Neighbors, friends, or fellow church or synagogue members might also be happy to pitch in and help with household chores or errands, if asked.

Emergency alert services are also available. Private or hospital-run companies provide twenty-four-hour service for a fee. Consumers wear an electronic device that can be activated in case of an emergency. This summons help to the wearer's home within a certain amount of time. This kind of service is particularly useful for someone who lives alone, but it shouldn't replace daily contact with friends or family. It is still a good idea to ask a neighbor to check in with you briefly. Or ask a "phone buddy" to give you a quick call each day—just to be sure everything is all right.

A different sort of alert system is available through the United States Postal Service. If asked, your post office representative will affix a red sticker to your mailbox, which alerts the carrier that you are disabled or have health problems. Then, if your mail isn't picked up from the day before, the carrier will alert a designated service agency to check and see whether you need help. Contact your local post office for more details.

Many local public libraries can provide a number of special services to their patrons. If you cannot get to the library yourself, many branches are happy to pick out books for you and deliver them to your home. For those who have difficulty reading, many books are available on tape.

Vocational Services

You may not be able to return to the job you had before your stroke, but there may be other work you'd like to do to remain active. Every state in the country has an Office of Vocational Rehabilitation, organized to help those who qualify find a job. To qualify, you must demonstrate to a counselor that you have either a disability that prevents you from working or financial need.

If you qualify, a counselor will design an individualized program for you. You may be referred to another agency for a job-training evaluation or an educational program. After that, the counselor will work with you to find you a job.

Contact your state Office of Vocational Rehabilitation for further information.

Financial Services

Private insurance carriers or federal and state agencies will pay for many hospital costs. Long-term care after a hospital stay, however, may require making special financial arrangements. A social worker can help you investigate potential sources of aid.

Your local area or state office on aging can help in a number of ways. You may be able to apply for food stamps, medical insurance, or financial aid through this office. In addition, you may be able to arrange for home health care, nursing, special equipment, transportation to doctor appointments, rehabilitation therapy, or day care.

Medicaid is an agency that helps pay for many medical needs associated with stroke described above, if you are eligible. Eligibility requirements vary among states and depend upon your income and savings. Benefits vary also.

Medicaid payments are made directly to the doctor or service provider, not to you. So don't pay for services expecting to be reimbursed by Medicaid later.

Medicare is a different program entirely. You are eligible for certain home health care benefits if you are over sixty-five and have been disabled for at least two years, regardless of your financial status. In general, Medicare will pay for short-term, skilled home health services. These might include: occasional, part-time, skilled nursing; physical therapy, speech therapy, and/or some occupational therapy; and some kinds of social work. Doctors' services and some special equipment are also covered. Long-term nursing maintenance isn't covered, except in a few states.

After you pay a deductible for the calendar year, Medicare will pay for a certain percentage of all "reasonable charges" of the services that they cover. For example, if Medicare pays 80 percent, you pay 20 percent of all "reasonable charges." You also pay 100 percent of anything that is "not reasonable" or not covered.

For more information about Medicare, contact your local Social Security office, or the Office of Health and Human Services in Washington, D.C.

You may want to look into special equipment coverage. Necessary equipment, such as wheelchairs, canes, ramps, and the like, may be covered under your insurance policy. Medicare and Medicaid will pay for all or some of these costs if the equipment has been prescribed by a doctor.

Private insurance companies vary widely. Each sets its type of coverage and amount of deductible. Read your policy closely and contact the company for more information.

Legal Services

If you have a legal problem and can't afford to pay a private attorney, there are places to go for help. Major cities usually have a Legal Aid Society office or some other government-funded legal agency. Government-funded legal services will take on problems you may have with your landlord. They will also look into problems you may have with other government agencies or programs, such as Medicare, Medicaid, Social Security, Supplemental Security Income, or food stamps.

Smaller towns and rural areas may also offer free legal services to those who qualify. Contact your county American Bar Association to locate the agencies that can help you.

Independence

When you come home from the hospital, your efforts are focused on returning to the greatest degree of independence possible. Often this requires facing some new challenges if there are physical, cognitive, or behavioral deficits. New habits and skills may be needed. These take time to learn and become comfortable with.

Most stroke survivors can make a lot of progress in their goals—often more than they had thought possible. Patience, effort, an optimistic attitude, and the support of family and friends make it possible.

Even though independence is an important goal, it shouldn't be your only goal. Preventing a second stroke should be a twin priority. It is to that effort that we turn our attention next.

8

Lifestyle and the Stroke Prevention Connection

Whether you've had a stroke or a TIA, chances are you have begun to look at the probable causes of your illness. You want to know how to reduce the likelihood of having another stroke in the future. That's as it should be. Identifying risk factors and working with your doctor to change your habits and improve your health are both very important. In fact, they are two of the most powerfully important parts of any complete treatment program for stroke.

The true risk of having a second stroke is different for every person. But certain averages may be helpful. If they follow the same lifestyle as before, most people who have had one stroke have about a 10 to 12 percent chance in each subsequent year of having another. This same group also has about a 5 percent chance of having a heart attack or dying in the same time period. Taken together, these odds suggest that the average stroke survivor has roughly a 15 to 17 percent chance per year of having one of these events. That's not good news, obviously. But is there any better news? Yes, absolutely.

The good news is, these percentages aren't nearly as high for those who, after a stroke, become actively involved in their own health care, take medications as prescribed, and change their contributing risk factors as much as possible. (Stroke risk factors are discussed fully in Chapter Two.) They reduce their risk of having another stroke by half. That's a 97 percent chance of *not* having a second stroke.

One preventive step might be long-term drug therapy to control high blood pressure or diabetes. Changing eating habits to bring down a high blood cholesterol level, stopping smoking, or having surgery may also be indicated. Each of these steps can help reduce or eliminate some stroke survivors' risk factors.

In this chapter, we'll look at ways a stroke survivor can learn to change some risk factors that fall within his control, such as diet, exercise, and smoking. Chapter Two explains more fully why it can be very important to make such changes. You may wish to review that chapter and discuss your particular risk factors with your doctor. He can put together a prevention plan that is best for you. If he doesn't discuss prevention with you, be persistent. Ask him what you can do to help prevent a second stroke.

Most of the risk factors that each of us can control are considered secondary, rather than primary, risk factors. (Smoking is an exception. It is a primary risk factor that we *can* control.) The term "secondary risk factor" means that poor habits in these areas do not cause strokes in themselves. However, they are linked to other very serious health problems, such as atherosclerosis or heart disease, that do contribute directly to stroke. Secondary risk factors often contribute to a variety of other life-threatening diseases. For this reason, controlling or eliminating them should be a serious goal for all health-minded individuals.

Ira was giving a doctor his full attention for the first time in his life. He had survived a brain hemorrhage, and now his doctor was telling him what he needed to do to reduce his risk of ever having a second stroke.

"As you now know, Ira," Dr. Shaw was saying, "having a stroke is in itself a warning sign for stroke—so you can't be too careful. You were extraordinarily lucky not to have had any more serious deficits than a slight hitch in your step. But I want you to be sure you take care of yourself from here on. OK?"

Ira nodded. He was waiting for the doctor to say something about his high blood pressure. He had known he had high blood pressure for years, but he just never did anything about it.

"I'm putting you on medication for your hypertension, Ira, and I want you to tell me you will take it faithfully. It is no joke—high blood pressure is a killer. Do we understand each other?"

Did he! Ira had heard almost nothing else from Dr. Shaw and his associates since he'd been in the hospital. "Yes, I know it's important. And I'll take it exactly as you prescribe it. I'll just get used to it."

"Good. Now, I'm giving you medication because your blood pressure is particularly high. But I want you to monitor the situation in two other ways also. The first is by watching the salt in your diet. A high-sodium diet can contribute to hypertension, so I'm giving you a balanced, nutritional, low-fat, low-salt diet right now that I want you to follow. Look at the back of the booklet. It lists the foods I want you to avoid completely —very salty, fatty things, like green olives, potato chips, that sort of thing. If you'd like more help with this, I can give you the name of an excellent nutritionist here at the hospital who would be glad to help you with your diet goals."

"I think I can manage that sort of diet. Just don't put me on one of those salads-only diets," Ira replied.

"The other thing I want you to start doing is get a little exercise. Now, relax! I'm not talking about climbing Mount Fuji on your weekends, or anything like that. I just want you to get some regular exercise three times a week for about thirty minutes a pop. Here's a pamphlet that explains which exercises are best for which benefits. Find something you like to do— maybe walking the dog or swimming. Lots of my patients walk around the enclosed mall downtown early in the morning. It's become quite the thing to do, I hear."

"I'll try, Doc."

"What I want to emphasize to you, Ira, is that lifestyle changes you make now can be very important to your health for the rest of your life. The exercise and diet changes I've suggested *can* help lower your blood pressure. They can also be good for your heart and lower your blood cholesterol level, too."

It all sounded pretty reasonable, Ira had to admit. And maybe he could get Bernice to walk the mall with him. That could be fun. Walking with his wife in a big air-conditioned mall didn't sound so bad.

"I want you to take these materials with you and read over them. Work on the lifestyle changes we talked about. Then come in and see me in two months. Any questions?" The doctor was finally winding down.

"Just one. Will it really make a difference—me making all these changes at age sixty-two?" Ira asked.

"Definitely. You're never too old to benefit from a healthy lifestyle. We'll see how you're doing in two months. Good luck, Ira. You can do it."

"I'll sure try."

The Importance of Practicing Prevention

Many of us grew up thinking health care was a resource to turn to only after we became ill. But today we know better. Many of the personal choices we make throughout our lives have a great deal to do with the kind of health we enjoy. By working as a partner with our health care practitioners, we can learn to practice the kind of healthful living that can prolong life. Eating wisely, being physically active, and not smoking are good ideas for everyone. So are having regular checkups and controlling medical problems. All of these can contribute positively to stroke prevention and to general good health.

The suddenness of stroke onset seems to suggest that this illness develops spontaneously. Actually, the reverse is true. As we've mentioned earlier in this book, stroke is generally the result of a lifetime of insults to the body. Fortunately, if the habits that caused those injuries are changed, the body benefits.

Sometimes, of course, people do go on to have second strokes, despite good health habits. But often their strokes are less serious than they might have been.

There has been a gradual change in the type and severity of stroke doctors diagnose in patients. That's because better health habits have caught on. Controlling high blood pressure, the most important risk factor for hemorrhagic stroke, is a good case in point. Doctors see fewer instances of hemorrhagic stroke these days. And the strokes they do see tend to be smaller and less damaging for those who have controlled their high blood pressure.

The brain is such a delicate instrument that even the slightest brain injury has serious consequences. Medical breakthroughs involving stroke care will continue to be made in the future. These will provide new hope for stroke survivors. But doctors agree that the very best way to treat stroke is to practice prevention. That is, stop a stroke *before* it happens, rather than repair the brain afterward.

Every stroke survivor can do a lot to reduce his chances of a second episode. And a person who has had a TIA can do a lot to reduce his chances of having a full-blown stroke. No one is "too old" to benefit from a sensible health plan, tailored to individual needs. Even for lifelong smokers and people who have neglected a medical condition for some time, there is hope. Stopping smoking or controlling the medical condition—starting now—*will* improve health. Doing these things will also reduce the risk of premature death or serious illness.

If you have had a stroke or a TIA, your doctor may urge you to make certain changes in your lifestyle. He may decide that you need special drug therapy to treat an underlying condition related to your stroke. Let's look at some of those areas now. You'll see why following your doctor's advice to the letter is good medicine for you.

Living with High Blood Pressure

Remember that hypertension—high blood pressure—is the major risk factor associated with stroke. It is perhaps the single most important preventable cause of stroke. Hypertension and its relation to stroke are discussed at length in Chapter Two. People with uncontrolled high blood pressure have a much greater risk than others of strokes, heart attacks, and other life-threatening illnesses.

Scientists don't know what causes hypertension in most cases. Most people with the condition cannot be cured of it. Fortunately, as serious as hypertension is, it is generally easy to identify and control.

A Team Effort

If you have high blood pressure, controlling it is a team effort. The team is composed of you, your doctor, and sometimes a registered dietitian or licensed nutritionist. (Friends and family should be your cheerleaders and lend you support.) Your doctor is the captain of your team. She will provide you with medical advice and instructions that will guide you in your effort. It's very important that you follow her instructions precisely. If you are confused about your doctor's instructions, ask questions until you understand. Dietitians or nutritionists can evaluate your eating habits and help you change them. They will take your high blood pressure and any other special needs into account.

Your job is to remain actively aware of your condition and to work at keeping your blood pressure within the appropriate range. Ask your doctor what your goal blood pressure level is and how soon you should reach it. Discuss whether home measurement would be a good idea for you. If it is, be sure you are properly trained by a professional to take accurate measurements. Keep a personal log of your blood pressure readings (see the chart on page 257).

Ask your doctor if you need any laboratory tests. If you do, ask what the tests are meant to show. Also ask if and when you should phone the office for the results.

Pay attention to the way you feel as the therapy goes on. If you feel different than usual, discuss it with your doctor. Remember, don't be afraid to ask your doctor plenty of questions. The more you know, the better you can follow directions.

Lifestyle Changes

Your doctor may ask you to make some changes in your lifestyle. Often, changing your lifestyle habits alone will be all that is needed to control an abnormally high blood pressure condition.

Eating Habits

Because high levels of sodium in the blood can contribute to a hypertension problem, your doctor may put you on a low-salt diet. (Table salt is about half sodium.) If you are overweight, which also contributes to hypertension, you may go on a slimming diet as well. Your doctor may give you a diet to follow, or refer you to a dietitian or nutritionist. (For more information on diets, see pages 251–261.)

Salt *alone* probably doesn't elevate one's blood pressure to abnormal levels. But if you have a predisposition to the condition, cutting back on salt in your diet can be a great tool for controlling hypertension. Your body gets all the sodium it needs naturally from the foods you eat. You don't need any added salt or sodium. So it's best to try to avoid table salt and processed foods with added salt or sodium. Concentrate instead on using fresh, canned, or frozen fruits and vegetables without added salt. Try low-fat meats that you can prepare simply yourself. Try grilling, poaching, or stir-frying, for example, rather than deep-frying. Try to avoid heavy sauces.

Check the content labels on the prepared foods you buy, and avoid those that are high in sodium. The obvious ones are salty snack-food items. You'll find the word *salt* on these labels. Often, however, some form of sodium is used in processing food. So, you also need to look for the word *sodium* on the label. These "hidden" sources of sodium in foods are a little harder to spot. Some examples are: **monosodium glutamate (MSG),** a flavor enhancer; **sodium bicarbonate,** a leavening agent; **sodium nitrite,** a meat preserver; **sodium benzoate,** a preservative; and **sodium citrate,** an acidity controller.

Also, check out the order in which the word *salt* or *sodium* appears on the ingredients list. This is a less precise way to evaluate how salty a packaged product is, but it can be helpful in some cases. Ingredients lists are organized according to the relative amounts of the ingredients that appear in the product. The ingredient that is first on the list is present in the greatest quantity. The rest of the ingredients are listed in descending order. The less salt or sodium the product contains, the farther down the list it will appear.

Some packaged products may make claims about the amount of sodium they contain as part of the sales pitch for the product.

These can be confusing for consumers, because of course all such claims attempt to make the product sound good. The following list describes current definitions for these terms:

Sodium free. The product contains less than 5 milligrams of sodium per serving.

Very low sodium. The product contains 35 milligrams or less per serving.

Low sodium. The product contains 140 milligrams or less per serving.

Reduced sodium. The product uses at least 25 percent less sodium than would be present in the food it replaces.

Unsalted, no salt added, and *without added salt* all mean that the product is made without the salt that is normally used. But remember that the food itself may still contain some sodium naturally.

When you first go on a low-salt diet, you may miss the flavor of salt. But don't despair. You can cultivate other tastes. Let yourself go—be creative! Experiment with herbs and spices in your cooking, instead of relying on salt. Substitute a sodium-free but flavorful seasoning blend for salt in your former salt shaker as well. Some of these blends are available commercially; some you can mix easily yourself.

Your doctor may recommend restricting alcoholic beverages if you have high blood pressure. Drinking more than two alcoholic drinks a day contributes to a hypertensive condition and makes it more difficult to control. (For specific recommendations, see pages 72 and 288.)

Exercise Habits

The relationship between exercise and high blood pressure isn't precisely known. It is believed, however, that a regular exercise program can help maintain a lower blood pressure level. Before you begin any exercise program, *be sure to get your doctor's permission.* Your blood pressure must be under control *before* starting any program. Your doctor may also recommend a fitness test before you begin to exercise.

NONSALTY SEASONING BLENDS

Try replacing the salt on your table with something flavorful and new. Here are some ideas to get you started.

Asian seasonings. Five-spice powder: 1 teaspoon ground cinnamon; 1 teaspoon crushed anise seed OR 1 star anise, ground; ¼ teaspoon fresh-ground pepper; ¼ teaspoon ground cloves; ¼ teaspoon crushed fennel seed. Mix together and store in an airtight container.

Cajun seasonings. Red, white, and black pepper; paprika; basil; thyme; and garlic.

Italian seasonings. Oregano, rosemary, basil, garlic, thyme, sage, and fennel.

Mexican seasonings. Cumin, cilantro, garlic, basil, cayenne pepper, and oregano.

Medications

Lifestyle changes alone may not be enough to bring your blood pressure down. Or your blood pressure may be so high that immediate steps are needed to bring it down to within the normal range. In either case, your doctor may prescribe medications for this purpose.

Follow your doctor's instructions for taking medications exactly. Be informed about what you are taking and why you are taking it. Find out the following information from your doctor—about your blood pressure medication as well as any other prescribed medication you may be taking.

- The name of the medication and what it's supposed to do.
- How often to take it.
- How much to take.
- How long to take it.
- How to store it. (Does the medication need to be stored in a cool place?)
- If there is a specific time of day it should be taken.
- If there are foods, drinks, other medications, or activities to avoid while on this medication (or any other precautions to take).

- What results, reactions, or side effects you might expect from the medication and what to do if you experience any.
- If there is any written information you can have to help you remember important points about the medication.
- What to do in case you miss a dose.
- How the medication affects pregnancy or breast-feeding.
- What to do if you get sick from something else or have to go the hospital. (Should you continue to take the medication?)

You may want to keep a small notebook in which to jot down questions that you may think of between visits to the doctor. (You may also want to use it to take down notes and instructions during your appointment.)

Sometimes you may not have the chance to ask all the questions you wanted to during your examination. Or you may have forgotten your questions during the exam or just thought of them afterward. If you have any questions after you have dressed, be sure to ask to speak with your doctor before you leave. Always try to arrange for your next appointment before you leave the doctor's office. Or call the office as soon as you can to set up that appointment.

Smoking: Be a Quitter

Smoking, as Chapter Two established, is a primary risk factor for stroke. It is also a risk factor for a number of other medical hazards, including cancer, heart disease, high blood pressure, and atherosclerosis. Fortunately, that strong message is getting through to more and more Americans. In 1987 more than one-fourth of all American adults called themselves *former* smokers. In 1990 the percentage of Americans who still smoked was at an all-time low: 25 percent. But, of course, that percentage is still 25 percent too high. About 430,000 to 467,000 premature deaths per year are attributed to smoking. That's close to half a million avoidable deaths every year. Unfortunately, that fact is hidden behind sophisticated ads that promote cigarette smoking as somehow glamorous.

If you have had a stroke or TIA and still smoke, stop and think for a moment. You have had one of the strongest possible warnings that you must stop smoking immediately. Stroke is a frightening, terrible experience—but it also may be the most important motivation for quitting you will ever have. Use it! Quitting smoking still won't be easy, of course. But the health benefits of doing so probably will mean more to you—and your loved ones—than ever before. And you'll find that's a powerful incentive. People who stop smoking slow down the development of atherosclerosis in their carotid arteries. The risk of death or heart attack drops for those with existing heart disease. And there are other health benefits as well (which are reviewed in Chapter Two).

J.D. was in a very bad mood. Not only had he had a stroke the week before, but now he was stuck in the hospital. To top it all off, it looked like he would have to quit smoking. As he brooded on the situation, J.D.'s doctor appeared at his bedside.

"Good morning, J.D.," Dr. Tedesco said cheerfully. "How do you feel today?"

"I feel lousy, thank you very much. I want a cigarette badly. I still don't see how my smoking and my stroke are connected, Doc."

"Well, they are connected through your cardiovascular system. You had an embolic stroke that technically was caused by atrial fibrillation in your heart. That means that your heart wasn't pumping effectively. Some of your blood pooled in one of the chambers instead of being pumped out into the bloodstream like it was supposed to be. When the blood was allowed just to sit there, it clotted. Some little clots were eventually swept out into the bloodstream. Some dissolved and some got stuck in vessels. You had a stroke because at least one embolism got stuck in a blood vessel in your brain."

"Sounds to me like it was my heart not working right. What does that have to do with smoking?" J.D. asked.

Dr. Tedesco sat on a nearby chair and continued. "Let's

back up to the cardiovascular system again. Your cigarette smoking affects your lungs, blood, and heart profoundly. By smoking, you introduce more than four thousand foreign elements into your bloodstream through the lungs. These get carried through the bloodstream, scraping the blood vessels as they go by. We suspect that over time this injures the blood vessels. Your blood has to carry the carbon monoxide from the smoke into the body instead of the oxygen it's supposed to carry. But the body still needs the oxygen, so the heart has to pump a little harder to try to make up the difference. That probably wears down the heart a bit faster, too. And finally, all those foreign elements in the blood may contribute to a thick-blood problem. That may encourage blood clotting and the formation of emboli in its own right. So you see, while there may be no direct link between smoking and your stroke, we have plenty of evidence to prove that smoking is strongly associated with the mechanisms involved in stroke. We aren't guessing here. *You really must not smoke ever again.*"

"But I feel like I really need a cigarette—with all this stress."

"J.D., I promise you will lose this very intense craving for nicotine."

J.D. loved smoking, but he knew he never wanted to go through anything as scary as a stroke ever again, either. So he resolved not to smoke when he was released from the hospital. He'd sure miss it, though.

Three months later, J.D. saw his doctor for a checkup. Dr. Tedesco asked if he had been smoking.

"Not once, Doc," J.D. said proudly. "And you know, it was pure agony not to. I know I'll always miss it. But something great has happened. One morning, I had a glass of orange juice, just like always. But it was the greatest orange juice I'd ever tasted! I can't even describe how good it was. I told my wife to try it. She took a sip and said it tasted like it always did. That's when it hit me: I was really tasting it for the first time in years! That was quite a feeling, let me tell you."

"How do you feel?" Dr. Tedesco asked.

"Better every day. I'm coughing less, and I have a little more energy. I still get tired—especially after physical therapy. But I'm breathing better. It's really great to have something positive like this to think of when the urge to smoke hits. No way am I ever going back to that dirty habit. No way!"

Of course, no one can make a smoker quit. You must be ready to do it yourself. You must be committed to the effort and prepared to stick with it for the long haul. Having had a stroke, you may feel more than ready to quit. But you may not be sure how to do it, once and for all.

A Four-Point Plan to Stop Smoking

To stop smoking permanently is hard, no doubt about it. But it is *not* impossible. You'll need plenty of determination to succeed, and you'll need a concrete plan. The support of your friends and family will be very important, too. Enlist their aid before you start. At the same time, seek out the guidance of your doctor or a professional counselor. He will know a lot about what you are trying to accomplish and will be an excellent source of information and support as you work to reach your goal. A support group, in which ex-smokers meet regularly to talk about their experiences, can be helpful, too. Your local hospital may be able to direct you to one.

Many successful ex-smokers have followed this four-point plan to kick their habit:

1. *Identify the habit.* Like many other habitual activities, smoking is something you can wind up doing a lot of without ever really thinking about it. Before you attempt to quit, know what your habit really is. Be clear about how much you smoke every day and when. You also need to know the emotional or situational triggers that make you desire a cigarette. Knowing your enemy well now will help you defeat it later. Keep a record of your smoking activities in a small notebook until you are familiar with your smoking urges.

   Ask your doctor or counselor to suggest techniques to help you modify your behavior. He may provide you with a formal behavior modification strategy. This can help you substitute healthier behaviors for smoking when a trigger situation arises. Some doctors prescribe certain medical therapies for smokers. Two of these, skin patches and nicotine gum, are discussed briefly below.

2. *Identify the reasons for stopping smoking—forever.* Obviously, the fact that you've had a stroke or TIA is probably the best motivation for quitting there is. But don't stop there. Think of other reasons—there are so many. Review the section on smoking in Chapter Two of this book about risk factors. Take a look at the box on page 250 that lists some immediate benefits of quitting.

   Talk to others who have successfully quit. Think of people who have wanted you to quit and will be proud of you. Make a list of all these personal reasons. Then post them where you can see them often, such as on your refrigerator or desk.

   Most people do gain some weight after they stop smoking, although usually not much. Discuss this possibility with your doctor in advance if it worries you.

3. *Choose a "quit day."* This will be your liberation day—the day you are freed from smoking forever. Prepare for it, and make the mental commitment to your new, more healthful life, which will begin on that day.

4. *Follow up with the doctor.* See your doctor (or professional counselor) soon after your declared quit day to check on your progress. (Make that appointment before you quit.) Discuss any questions or anxieties and make any adjustments to your program at this time. If you're doing fine, give yourself a pat on the back—and keep going! Before you leave the office, make further checkup appointments as you and your doctor find it necessary.

Aids to Quitting

Some people benefit from taking prescribed drugs while they try to quit smoking. Your doctor can discuss them in detail with you. Two common ones are discussed below.

THE JOYS OF QUITTING:
SOME IMMEDIATE BENEFITS WHEN YOU STOP SMOKING

1. You'll be able to breathe better.
2. You'll regain your sense of smell.
3. You'll regain your sense of taste.
4. You'll save money.
5. You'll need less sleep.
6. You'll have more energy.
7. Your breath will be fresher.
8. Your environment won't smell of smoke.
9. No more ashtrays to empty.
10. No more burn holes.
11. You'll cut your risk of death by fire by 50%.
12. No more tobacco stains on your teeth and fingers.
13. You'll decrease risks of passive smoking for family and coworkers.
14. You'll be more employable.
15. You'll become a better insurance risk and enjoy cheaper insurance premiums.
16. Your lungs will be able to cleanse themselves better.
17. You'll have better coronary and peripheral circulation.
18. Your heart rate will go down.
19. You'll have lower blood carbon monoxide levels.
20. You'll perspire less.
21. You'll be able to exercise better.
22. You'll be able to do more physical work.
23. You'll have lower grocery bills.
24. You'll have extra time.
25. You'll get less social pressure from people who don't like your smoking habit.

Adapted, with permission, from the *Journal of General Internal Medicine,* 1988.

Usually nicotine gum is prescribed for smokers who are worried about excessive weight gain after they stop. Nicotine gum is not for everyone. It has drawbacks, among which are its expense and the fact that it continues the smoker's nicotine addiction. You must chew the gum slowly to release the nicotine steadily. If you drink coffee or soft drinks at the same time, you may reduce the gum's effectiveness.

Prescribed skin patches, which are worn on the upper arm, have become available only recently as a means of combatting a smoking habit. There is still some controversy over the true effectiveness of these skin patches for helping a smoker quit. Moreover, it is dangerous to wear the patch if you continue to smoke. So check with your doctor first.

Diet and Common Diet Problems

More and more scientific evidence is uncovered every day to back up the old maxim, "You are what you eat." Diet—proper nutrition—plays an important part in your overall health. Whether you eat too much of the wrong things—such as salty or fatty foods—or just too much altogether, the message is clear. The nutritional imbalances that result can adversely affect your health over time. Too much sodium in the diet can contribute to high blood pressure in many individuals. Eating too much fat in your regular diet can spur the development of high blood cholesterol and atherosclerosis. Obesity—defined as being 30 percent or more above one's ideal weight—is associated with a number of health problems. All of these adverse dietary conditions translate into risk factors for stroke.

Your doctor may have determined that one of these conditions has contributed to your stroke profile. She may want you to go on a special diet to correct it. If your doctor gives you a diet, be sure to follow it closely. If the diet you select did not come from your doctor, be sure she approves of it.

"Evelyn, we're going to work together on this so you can reduce your chances of having another stroke, OK?" Dr. Ringwald was talking to her patient Evelyn, who was in the hospital after having a mild stroke.

Evelyn was ready to listen. At sixty-three, she had already had a number of TIAs before finally being felled by a full-blown, though minor, stroke. She had ignored the warning signs because she hadn't known what they meant. Besides, they always just went away. But here she was in the hospital.

The doctor described a three-front attack. Evelyn's weight was too high. At five-foot-three she weighed 210 pounds. She would definitely have to lose weight. She had high blood pressure, for which she would need to take medication. Finally, her blood cholesterol level was also somewhat elevated. Like her blood pressure, that would need to be reduced also.

"The good news is that all of these things are interrelated," Dr. Ringwald said. "By following the diet I give you, you'll not only lose weight but also reduce your cholesterol level and help lower your blood pressure, too."

Evelyn was apprehensive. She knew how hard dieting could be, and she wasn't looking forward to it at all. She was sixty-three! What was really realistic for her at this point? she wondered.

"That's a tall order, Doctor," Evelyn remarked.

"I don't expect you to look the way you did when you were seventeen. This diet is not designed for that, Evelyn. It's not a beauty diet; it's a health diet. I think we can reasonably expect you to lose fifty pounds. You can also lower your cholesterol level and your blood pressure. But most important, I think you'll feel better and eat a better range of foods by following this diet. I want you to check in with me periodically and we'll see how you're doing. If you'd like, I can get you into a diet support group that meets once a week at the hospital, too."

Evelyn stuck with it. She took her medicine for high blood pressure faithfully. She followed the diet her doctor had recommended and joined the support group as well.

A year later, Evelyn had reached all of her goals and was in much better health than she had been in years. Her blood pressure and serum cholesterol levels were well within normal ranges, and she had dropped fifty-seven pounds through sensible, careful eating. She even walked regularly for exercise now, joined often by some of the friends she had made at her diet support group.

When Dr. Ringwald saw Evelyn again, she was pleased with her patient's success. She decided to take Evelyn off the high blood pressure medication as an experiment. When Evelyn's blood pressure stayed within normal range, Dr. Ringwald kept her off. Apparently Evelyn's new weight, diet, and exercise took care of the problem adequately.

"Way to go, Evelyn!" Dr. Ringwald said.

Choosing a Diet

Everyone should follow a healthful eating plan, although not everyone needs to lose weight. Others, because of some health condition, may need to follow a diet that restricts certain foods. People with high blood pressure may be on low-salt diets. People with high blood cholesterol may be on low-fat, low-cholesterol diets. Still others with chewing and swallowing difficulties may be on diets restricted to certain types of food.

A good diet is well balanced and contains adequate fiber, much of which is found in foods containing complex carbohydrates. Sadly, the typical American diet is not as healthful as it should be. Most Americans consume too much sodium from prepared foods and get more calories from fat than they should. A good diet has less than 30 percent of calories from fat. Americans on average consume 37 percent of their daily calories from fat.

A doctor or registered dietitian can help you put together an appropriate diet plan. So can the American Heart Association. Our suggested basic diet is reprinted in the Appendix section of this book (pages 279–289). Bear in mind that while it is a naturally low-fat and low-sodium diet, it may not be as restrictive as your doctor may wish for you. You may require a different diet if you need to lose weight or control hypertension, for example. Before beginning any new diet, check with your doctor to make sure you have chosen the diet that is most suitable for your needs.

Motivation and Planning

Changing what might be called a "style" of eating isn't easy. After all, most of us have been "perfecting" our own for years! But with proper preparation, permanent change is possible. Planning and motivation are perhaps the most important keys to success with any kind of diet.

Before starting a diet, be very clear about the reasons you are undertaking the enterprise. Your motivation is very important. Only you can motivate yourself to lose excess weight or otherwise significantly change your eating habits. Obviously, the fact that you've had a stroke or a TIA is an extremely strong motivator for sticking with a diet (and losing excess weight, if necessary). Other motivations may be to gain more control over your life in general or to look or feel better.

Motivation is perhaps the element most critical to the success of any long-term change in eating patterns. But planning and preparation are important to keep you on track. Planning and preparation also will help you meet potentially high-risk situations. They will help you handle dinner parties and other occasions more confidently. Be prepared before starting your diet. Think about what you want to accomplish and how you plan to achieve your goals. Talk with others about your plans. Doing so can help you articulate your goals. Make the mental commitment to this worthwhile lifestyle change before you begin, and visualize all the benefits of sticking with the program.

You might follow a menu plan, enlist the support of friends and family, or try behavior modification techniques. You might also incorporate an appropriate exercise program into your life. For most people, such a multidisciplinary program works best, both to reach their goals and to maintain them.

Behavior Modification

Behavior modification helps some dieters, especially those who are trying to lose excess weight and keep it off. Many dieters keep a detailed record, or diary, about what they eat during the day. They also note when they eat and how they feel at the time. They use this to help recognize certain "triggers" in their daily routine that prompt them to eat or to crave the wrong foods—such as sugary, salty, or fat-laden snacks.

Some may learn, for example, that they are likely to eat certain kinds of food when they are feeling anxious or depressed. Others may realize that they unconsciously reach for food when they are in certain rooms or doing certain activities, such as watching TV in the evening. Some may find they don't enjoy cooking in the evening. Instead, they rely on high-fat, high-sodium prepared foods that are easy to fix quickly.

The importance of keeping a diary is to teach dieters to be aware of their behavior and to recognize the signals that may encourage overeating or eating the wrong foods. Once they recognize these triggers, they can compensate for them in some other way. Looking at the diary also helps a diet counselor identify these trouble spots and devise ways around them. The person who eats because she is anxious might instead substitute a walk around the block, a shower, or fifteen minutes of concentrated listening to favorite music. The person who reaches for food every time she sits down in front of the TV might decide to eat in just one room, such as the dining room. And the person who eats fast food because she is too tired to cook at night might experiment with simple dishes prepared in advance. These dishes can be made from scratch at any time and then divided into servings and frozen or refrigerated. They can then be warmed up quickly later in the week.

During Your Diet

You may be following a diet to lose weight, to bring down your cholesterol levels, or to control your blood pressure. Or your diet goal may combine all three. Whatever your diet goal, there are many ways to maximize your success. Three of these are discussed below.

Find Some Cheerleaders

Changing lifelong eating habits does not happen overnight. Your effort deserves the positive support of your friends and family. Don't be isolated as you work on this exciting challenge. Let others know your plans to change your eating habits. Tell them how you will be going about it and how they can help you achieve your goals. Ask them to reinforce the positive habits you are trying to instill by not tempting you with the foods you want to avoid. Ask for their understanding of what you are trying to accomplish.

It can be very helpful to work at changing your eating patterns under the close supervision of your doctor or a registered dietitian or licensed nutritionist. Make this person your ally, and discuss any problems, temptations, or successes you have with him. These professionals are there to help. You can locate registered dietitians and licensed nutritionists through your hospital or your doctor.

Be Realistic

After a stroke, you may not be as active as you were before. As a result if you are on a slimming diet, it may take longer for you to lose weight. This is to be expected, so allow yourself plenty of time to reach your goal. Don't be hard on yourself if you think you aren't losing weight as quickly as you'd like. Slow but steady will get you there just fine.

Temptations will always be there. The key is to be ready for them before they present themselves. Family and friends may urge you to eat some foods you want to avoid. Plan ahead to respond to their temptations firmly and politely. Don't back down! You are under no obligation to accept food or to apologize for declining it.

You can plan ahead for other sticky spots as well. Parties, at which rich foods are often served, can be a problem for many. The solution is to eat a bulky, low-calorie snack just before going out. A crisp apple is a good choice. You'll be less likely to nibble on appetizers and be well satisfied with smaller portions of any high-calorie, rich dishes you may be served. You might feel that you will go off your diet at some of the usual places you go with friends. If so, try to meet them at new places that are less tempting for you instead.

Emotions as well as certain places or situations prompt many people to eat more or crave certain foods. You may learn that you tend to eat more or eat certain kinds of "indulgence foods" if you are happy, angry, worried, or depressed. By keeping a food diary (see the section on behavior modification on pages 254–255), you can learn to recognize these trigger situations and substitute other behaviors for eating when they occur.

On any diet, no one is perfect, and there will be times when you will have setbacks in your dieting program. If you have high blood pressure, for example, you may lapse and indulge a sudden craving for salty tastes. The important thing is not to give up. Be flexible and resolve to keep working to make your new eating habits permanent.

Plateaus are common in any diet, too. After losing a number of pounds consistently over the weeks, you may discover that your weight loss has slowed or leveled off. Or you may find your cholesterol level has become "stuck" for a while at a certain level, despite your efforts to lower it. This is natural and temporary, if a bit frustrating. Expect it—and keep going.

Finally, don't set impossible goals for yourself. Break the job into smaller, more manageable pieces. If your ultimate goal, for example, is to lose thirty pounds, concentrate on losing the first five pounds, and then the next, and so on.

It can help to keep a long-term record of your progress, perhaps in the form of a weight, blood pressure, or cholesterol level chart or graph. When you take the long view of your goal, it may put small slips into better perspective. Your goal, after all, is to make a permanent change in your eating habits. This takes time.

YOUR BLOOD PRESSURE, WEIGHT, AND BLOOD CHOLESTEROL RECORD

Your blood pressure goal _____

Your weight goal _____

Your blood cholesterol goal _____

Date	Blood Pressure	Weight	Blood Cholesterol

A Winning Combination

Combine your diet with an exercise program, if possible. Although not an option for all stroke survivors, exercise does increase one's daily energy needs. As a result, you burn more calories as fuel. An exercise habit can help you lose excess weight faster, and it can provide other benefits as well. For example, it can increase the HDL, or "good," cholesterol levels in the bloodstream. It also benefits your cardiovascular system, strengthening the heart. It helps you maintain your desired weight once you've achieved your goal. And it makes you feel good!

Note: Because you have had a stroke or TIA, check with your doctor before starting a regular exercise program. If you have high blood pressure, it must be brought down within a normal range *first.* Exercise is discussed more fully below (see pages 261–276).

What About Crash Diets?

To put it bluntly, quick-loss diets, also called "crash diets" or "fad diets," just don't work. Excess weight may come off quickly, as promised, but it also tends to reappear just as quickly—often with a few added pounds for good measure. Such diets are not only ultimately frustrating, but they can be dangerous to your health. Doctors recommend that you lose no more than about a pound or two a week for permanent weight loss.

A fad diet that depends on just a few foods or severely restricts foods has serious disadvantages. It can deprive you of important nutrients, and it won't teach you the kind of habits that you need to develop to keep the excess weight off. By eating regular, nutritious meals, your body will get all the nutrients it needs. And you can still achieve your personal goals.

Stay away from diets and programs that promise to help you lose weight—or solve any other problem—quickly. Slowly but surely is best. If your doctor believes you should follow a certain diet, remember that you are working on both short-term and long-term goals in this effort. First, you are trying to solve an immediate problem, such as being overweight or having high blood pressure. Second, you are relearning eating habits that will last a lifetime and result in better overall health. This is important whether you are trying to wean yourself from the taste of salt, trying to avoid sugary or high-cholesterol foods, or trying to lose excess weight. Along the way, you'll retrain your taste buds to prefer the flavors and textures of low-calorie foods instead of high-calorie ones, and you'll learn to judge how much food you really need.

In short, don't condemn yourself to so-called diet food. You'll feel deprived and be tempted to binge later. Diets should emphasize

DESIRABLE BODY WEIGHT RANGES

HEIGHT WITHOUT SHOES	WEIGHT WITHOUT CLOTHES	
	Men	Women
(feet/inches)	(pounds)	(pounds)
4'10"	—	92–121
4'11"	—	95–124
5'0"	—	98–127
5'1"	105–134	101–130
5'2"	108–137	104–134
5'3"	111–141	107–138
5'4"	114–145	110–142
5'5"	117–149	114–146
5'6"	121–154	118–150
5'7"	125–159	122–154
5'8"	129–163	126–159
5'9"	133–167	130–164
5'10"	137–172	134–169
5'11"	141–177	—
6'0"	145–182	—
6'1"	149–187	—
6'2"	153–192	—
6'3"	157–197	—

This table is adapted from the Desirable Weight Table prepared in 1959 by the Metropolitan Life Insurance Company. It is based on weights associated with the lowest mortality. For women 18 to 25 years, subtract one pound for each year under 25.

The 1983 revision of the Metropolitan Life Insurance Company's Height and Weight Tables allows increased weight for certain heights. However, because obesity is a contributing factor for heart disease, the American Heart Association did not adapt the 1983 version.

the same kinds of eating plans that everyone should follow. Eat a wide variety of foods. Include fruits, vegetables, skim milk, low-fat dairy products, cereals and grains, lean meats, fish, and poultry in limited amounts. Eat minimal amounts of margarine, vegetable oil, and salad dressings. Eat foods prepared with limited amounts of fat and salt. Make few high-calorie choices (such as fats, sugars, alcohol). Keep portions moderate.

It helps to shop well. Stock up on unprocessed food you can prepare yourself. Plan your meals and use a shopping list. Don't leave eating to chance, or you may be tempted to cheat. And don't go grocery shopping on an empty stomach.

After You Reach Your Goal

Congratulations! Maintaining your ideal blood pressure level, cholesterol level, or weight will have its own challenges. But it's nothing you can't handle. Here are some tips to help you maintain your new levels through diet.

- Add some calories to your daily diet after you reach your desired weight. Do this by adding nutritious low-fat foods. You might slowly increase servings of cereal, grains, fruits, and vegetables, for example. If you are still losing weight after a week at the new level, add some more calories. Then check your weight again in a week. Continue in this pattern until you stabilize at your ideal weight.
- If your exercise habits change, be sure to adjust your daily caloric intake accordingly.
- Keep a weekly chart of your weight and blood pressure levels, so you can respond to fluctuations before they can get out of hand. Discuss with your doctor how often your blood cholesterol levels should be checked.
- Snack sensibly, if at all. Between meals, drink water, low-fat or nonfat milk, iced or hot tea, or coffee. (Be aware, however, that your doctor may suggest that you limit your intake of caffeinated drinks such as tea and coffee, especially if you have a tendency to experience arrhythmias.) If you routinely get hungry during the day, reserve something from another meal to eat at that time. A piece of fruit saved from lunch is a good idea. Stay out of the kitchen if it isn't mealtime. Stay busy.
- Practice delayed gratification. When you are tempted to eat a snack you want to avoid, set a timer for fifteen minutes and tell yourself you'll eat then if you still

want to. Then do something else during that time. Chances are, you will find that the desire for the food subsides to a point at which you can resist it completely. Or you may substitute a lower-calorie snack, such as a piece of fruit or a tall glass of unsweetened iced tea, for what you had planned to eat originally.

- Handle cravings sensibly. The goal of lifelong good eating habits is not to deprive you permanently of foods you may still like. The goal is to put you in control of those likes. Once you have reached your goal, it is OK to occasionally eat a moderate portion of a favorite treat. But plan for it and stick within your overall calorie, sodium, or fat limits for that day. If you get a strong craving for something, try eating just a small amount. If you wait, you may gorge on it later instead. But if you find you can't handle a taste of something without eating a great deal—don't tempt yourself. Don't eat any at all.

- Substitute behavior. By substituting a different behavior for your old food dependency, you break the old cycle. If you usually reach for a bag of potato chips when you feel anxious, stop! Go for a different activity, like eating a crunchy carrot, going for a walk, reading, or bathing, instead.

- Learn to cope with "lapses, relapses, and collapses" in your eating habits. Don't consider what happened a failure—consider it a challenge that you will overcome. Identify the urges and high-risk situations that may be tempting you. Then, go back over the section on behavior modification (see pages 254–255) for help.

- Enjoy better health and increased vitality!

Exercise: The Experience of a Lifetime

Scientists have not found a direct link, good or bad, between regular exercise and stroke. But they do know that exercise reduces the risk of a variety of other health problems, such as heart disease, which can contribute to stroke.

Not all stroke survivors, of course, can or should engage in a vigorous exercise program. Abilities after a stroke vary greatly. Still, every person benefits from some type of regular activity. Depending upon the disabilities left by a stroke, exercise can be an important way of preventing complications associated with weakness or paralysis in the limbs or on one side of the body. For those with mild deficits, regular exercise can help strengthen muscles. It can also make the activities associated with independence—such as bathing and getting into and out of a chair—easier.

Peter was seventy-five years old. Never very active, he had become even less so after a stroke put him in a wheelchair late the year before. When asked about what kinds of activities he might like to do, he would laugh and say, "I'm an old professor. We like to exercise our eyes and read a lot!"

In the retirement community for academics where he lived, Peter was encouraged to join an exercise program that was just beginning. It was designed especially for people who were in wheelchairs. Peter could not imagine what this might be like. Out of curiosity, he decided to stop by. He was drawn to the room by the music. Four or five of his friends were already there, and they all urged him to join them. "It'll be fun," they said. "Or if not fun, at least different!"

But the class was fun. Peter became quite fond of the movements and the jazzy music. The instructor was a real professional, too; he liked that. The group learned to stretch and flex from a stationary position. Those who could would stand for some parts of the program, leaning against their chairs.

"I always feel more awake after this class," he remarked to his friend Bill after one session several weeks into the program. "I find it helps me concentrate better the rest of the day."

"You're hooked, Peter," Bill said. "I should know—I am, too!"

Check with your doctor before starting any exercise program. He will help you choose the kind of activity that is best suited to your individual condition. The point is to find some kind of helpful regular exercise that you are comfortable with. It can be stretching the arms and flexing the toes, walking around the block, or something else. Appropriate, regular exercise not only benefits the body, but it can brighten your outlook as well.

Obviously, an exercise program that makes sense for someone with severe deficits isn't likely to suit someone who has had a TIA and vice versa. Exercises for those who are more seriously impaired may emphasize stretching and flexibility. These exercises do not give the body's cardiovascular system (heart and lungs) a thorough workout. However, they are still very important. Done regularly, they can help keep the body limber, prevent cramping, and improve circulation to the limbs. Those with less severe physical or intellectual deficits might choose a more intense workout program —given the permission of their doctors, of course.

Start Right: Consult Your Doctor First

Because you've had a stroke or TIA, consult your doctor before starting any exercise program. Ask him about the types of exercise you might pursue safely and enjoyably. Many people equate the notion of exercise and personal fitness with jogging or some other equally active sport. In fact, fitness is a very personal matter, different for each of us according to our needs and abilities. Many stroke survivors, for example, may use some exercise time to work on strengthening muscle groups that allow them to stand without help. Your own exercise program should take your individuality into account. Your doctor or registered physical therapist can help tailor a worthwhile program just for you. Your progress should be monitored periodically by your doctor in the beginning.

Note: If you have high blood pressure, it must be brought under control before you start exercising.

Don't exercise too hard at the beginning of your program. Instead, follow a general, sound program in which you build up strength and endurance gradually. You should never feel winded, faint, or ill from exercise. If you do, slow down or stop. Take your time.

Feeling Good About Exercise

After a stroke, you may not feel as good as you did before. And you may look a little different, too. Exercise can't change the fact that you have had a stroke. But regular activity that is appropriate for

263

you can still improve your life in a number of ways. A regular exercise program can help you:

- feel more energetic;
- cope with stress better;
- resist fatigue better;
- counter feelings of anxiety and depression;
- relax more easily;
- fall asleep more easily at night and get better rest; and
- discover a pleasant way to spend time with friends and family and to make new friends.

Some Common Myths About Exercise

We've all heard that exercise is good for one's general health. But a lot of people resist the idea of getting regular exercise for "practical" reasons. Let's consider some of these common concerns.

1. *"I'm not a good enough athlete to exercise."* Many people think exercise takes special talents, but this isn't really true. A beneficial exercise program doesn't mean you have to be a star basketball player or a tennis ace. The simplest exercises can yield important benefits to those who practice them regularly. Some people who have had a stroke, for example, may focus on stretching exercises that can improve their balance or circulation.

2. *"It takes too much time, and I'm a busy person."* Some people fear that getting regular exercise is troublesome and will complicate their schedule. Actually, any activity is better than none. It's a good idea to exercise even if you can do very little at the beginning of your program. The optimal workout need not last more than one hour, three or four times a week. But shorter periods of exercise are also beneficial. Remember, it is better to be active than not active.

   Stretching exercises are best done every day for about fifteen minutes. Strengthening exercises are usually done every other day for an additional fifteen minutes. (Of course, for safety's sake, exercise only when you feel well and alert.) When you consider how much more time most of us spend every day watching television, this kind of an exercise schedule suddenly appears much more manageable. True, it may take a little getting used to at first. After you establish a regular routine, however, you'll find an exercise program fits quite naturally into your life. You may even feel deprived if you have to miss a session occasionally.

3. *"Exercise always makes me tired."* Many people put off exercising because they're afraid it will make them feel more tired than they are already. Actually, after you get used to it, you'll find the reverse is true. You'll gain more energy as a result of your exercise plan. Regular exercise also helps alleviate feelings of tension and fatigue. You'll feel more upbeat and alert.

4. *"Aren't I too old to exercise?"* It is a common misunderstanding that we need less exercise as we age. In fact, everyone needs to maintain an appropriate exercise level throughout life. Older people will find that exercise at an appropriate fitness level helps control high blood pressure and helps improve cardiovascular fitness. It also helps preserve bone density and adds to their life span. Exercise can improve your sense of balance, preventing falls. It can also help relieve constipation and help you sleep.

5. *"I can't exercise in a wheelchair."* There are many good exercise programs for people who use wheelchairs. A good exercise program can help every person be the best he can be.

Choosing the Right Exercise Program

Part of the long-term success of any exercise program depends on finding the right fit between you and a chosen activity. Don't assume that exercise has to be exhausting to be effective. That isn't the case. Stroke outcomes differ from one person to another. For some, concentrating on improving flexibility and balance are important goals. For others with greater mobility, developing a regular activity such as walking is a priority. Everyone, however, can benefit from some kind of regular program.

Answers to the following questions can help you identify appropriate activities you might enjoy:

- How physically fit are you? Consider any disabilities you may have.
- How old are you? Everyone benefits from exercise, but some activities may be more appropriate than others, depending upon one's age and ability.
- Do you like to exercise alone or with others? An exercise companion can help you stick with your program, especially in the beginning. Some exercises may require the assistance of another as well.
- Do you like to exercise outdoors or at home? Outdoors offers a change of scenery, but weather can pose a problem. (If you like to exercise outdoors, consider an alternative activity that you can perform indoors when the weather is poor.)
- How much money do you wish to spend on this activity? You don't have to spend a lot. Walking takes only an investment in a good pair of shoes. Your community's recreation department may also offer inexpensive exercise classes, or they may refer you to some.
- What's your schedule? Determine what your active times of day are, and fit in exercise around them. For best results, spread out your exercise program across the week. Every other day is good.

You also need to decide what benefits you want from an exercise program. Better flexibility? Improved heart rate? Ask your doctor to help you define your needs. Some activities condition the body's cardiovascular system (heart, lungs, and circulation). Less strenuous programs, however, are preferable for many stroke survivors. These programs yield important benefits, too. They might emphasize developing muscle flexibility and tone, for example. Your doctor can help you decide on a program that makes the most sense for you.

Exercises to Improve Flexibility and Muscle Tone

You and your doctor may choose for you an exercise program that improves flexibility and muscle tone and relieves stress. Activities in this category condition the heart very little, but almost everyone can do them. Often they do not involve sustained activity. You may not pursue them regularly. However, they can still provide certain benefits. They can improve coordination and body awareness, make joints more flexible (better range of motion), improve muscle tone, and give a sense of relaxation.

Stretching. Gentle stretching exercises fall into this category. They are often done to music. You can do them at home or in a class under an instructor's guidance. Talk to your physical therapist about options. Ask him about where to find classes, or ask at your community recreation center or stroke club. There are also videocassettes if you want to perform a routine at home. (If you choose to work out at home, you may need a "spotter"—someone who can physically support you for some positions or assist you if you run into difficulty with an exercise. This depends on your deficit level and is something to discuss with your doctor or registered physical therapist before you start.)

Stretching exercises may be done from a seated position. Wheelchairs (with the brakes on!) work fine. So do simple, sturdy chairs with a straight back, a firm seat, and armrests.

Do stretches only within your personal comfort level. Even small movements, done regularly and correctly, can be effective. Don't continue exercises that cause pain, discomfort, or fatigue. Wait to continue until the pain stops or you are stronger.

Stretches may involve the face, neck, shoulders, back, arms, hands, legs, feet, and even the trunk. Generally, the weak limb can be cradled or carefully lifted by the stronger one as you complete the exercises. In this way, both sides of the body are worked effectively, despite weakness or paralysis.

Deep, slow breathing is often a component of stretching exercise. Sometimes it is an exercise all by itself. Your physical therapist or stretch class instructor can discuss deep breathing with you. Deep, slow breathing can promote better oxygen exchange in the lungs, which is good for overall circulation. Inhaling and exhaling slowly and deeply can help reduce feelings of tension as well, which makes doing the exercises a bit easier and more enjoyable. Occasionally, slow, deep breathing causes dizziness or lightheadedness in some people. If this happens to you, stop immediately. And never go so far as to hold your breath while doing exercises.

Yoga. Yoga is an ancient art developed centuries ago in India. It combines very precise postures with deep breathing exercises, relaxation techniques, and stretching. It promotes a somewhat different concept of fitness that is gaining popularity in the United States. It may be an option for some people who have had a stroke.

Yoga can be a good form of exercise for a person who uses a wheelchair or who has physical deficits that prevent a more active exercise regime. As with any other exercise program, however, a doctor's approval is necessary before taking up yoga. Some postures, such as those that put the head below the heart for a period of time, are off-limits to some stroke survivors. A friend may be needed to provide assistance and support for some positions.

Yoga is good for improving one's sense of balance and positional awareness, as well as muscle strength. Its emphasis on serenity makes yoga a good choice for stress management and relaxation, too.

Easy Does It

Some people who have had a stroke are able to be a little more active. Many opportunities are available for them, with their doctor's approval. Many of these activities, if pursued regularly, can increase strength. They can also make it easier to perform other daily activities important to personal independence.

Strengthening Exercises. Strengthening exercises, done every other day, are a good idea for some. Some of the exercises below can be done from a wheelchair. Others require you to have good balance and be able to walk independently. Use sound judgment in selecting strengthening exercises appropriate for you. Exercises may start with warm-up stretches from a seated position and go on to a standing position. They may include partial knee bends, weight shifts, modified leg lifts, and the like.

Sometimes classes for these exercises are conducted in the shallow end of a swimming pool. This can be an especially attractive option if you have weakness or paralysis in some limbs. The water helps lift and support the weakened side in a natural way. The side of the pool provides support as well. (Knowing how to swim isn't necessary. However, the class should be taught by someone who has lifeguard training, or a lifeguard should be present.) You should feel securely balanced in the water at all times. Some people wear special socks with rubber soles for added protection against slipping.

Ask your physical therapist about where to find strengthening exercise classes. Or ask your doctor or physical therapist to recommend a videotape version to do at home. Be sure to have someone with you if your doctor recommends it, depending on your deficits.

Pleasure Walking. "Pleasure walking" is done at a moderate pace. Done regularly, it can help relieve stress, tone muscles, and increase energy. Walking is a popular choice for many stroke survivors with mild deficits. It can be done at one's own pace, alone or with others. About all it takes in the way of special equipment is a sturdy pair of shoes.

If you choose this form of exercise, be prepared to stretch adequately before every outing. Don't try to walk too far in the beginning. Start with a modest goal and gradually increase the amount you walk each day. A sample walking program developed by the American Heart Association appears on page 270. (The program as written may be too vigorous for some walkers who have had a stroke. So don't hesitate to establish your own goals in the place of those that have been suggested.) Choose a time of day that is good for you, and stick with it. Don't eat for a couple of hours before you go.

Walking can be done almost anywhere, of course, but it's a good idea to find a route that does not intersect with traffic, if possible. If you walk outdoors, have an alternative indoor route in mind for inclement days, such as the track in a community recreational center or school gym. More and more people are finding that their local indoor shopping mall is a great place to walk!

Other Ideas. Other activities in this category include gardening, yardwork, housework, bowling, golf, and softball. Be sure to ask your doctor or physical therapist to help you find a program that is right for *you.*

A SAMPLE WALKING PROGRAM

	Warm-up	Exercising	Cool-down	Total time
Week 1				
Session 1	Walk slowly 5 min.	Then walk briskly 5 min.	Then walk slowly 5 min.	15 min.
Session 2	Repeat above pattern.			
Session 3	Repeat above pattern.			
As long as you feel fine, exercise three times during each week of the program.				
Week 2	Walk slowly 5 min.	Walk briskly 7 min.	Walk slowly 5 min.	17 min.
Week 3	Walk slowly 5 min.	Walk briskly 9 min.	Walk slowly 5 min.	19 min.
Week 4	Walk slowly 5 min.	Walk briskly 11 min.	Walk slowly 5 min.	21 min.
Week 5	Walk slowly 5 min.	Walk briskly 13 min.	Walk slowly 5 min.	23 min.
Week 6	Walk slowly 5 min.	Walk briskly 15 min.	Walk slowly 5 min.	25 min.
Week 7	Walk slowly 5 min.	Walk briskly 18 min.	Walk slowly 5 min.	28 min.
Week 8	Walk slowly 5 min.	Walk briskly 20 min.	Walk slowly 5 min.	30 min.
Week 9	Walk slowly 5 min.	Walk briskly 23 min.	Walk slowly 5 min.	33 min.
Week 10	Walk slowly 5 min.	Walk briskly 26 min.	Walk slowly 5 min.	36 min.
Week 11	Walk slowly 5 min.	Walk briskly 28 min.	Walk slowly 5 min.	38 min.
Week 12	Walk slowly 5 min.	Walk briskly 30 min.	Walk slowly 5 min.	40 min.

More Vigorous Exercises

Note: Not all stroke survivors will be able to go beyond stretching and strengthening exercises. Some may, in time, move toward a more vigorous workout program of some kind. It really depends on your permanent deficits and general health after the stroke. Many exercise programs are just too vigorous for many stroke survivors. This includes those with significant deficits (such as trouble with vision, balance, or limb weakness) or other health concerns (such as atrial fibrillation). Check with your doctor first, of course.

Remember, every exercise level has its own virtues and rewards. And every person has his own individual exercise needs and capabilities. The old adage "No pain, no gain" is obsolete today. The point is *not* to do the toughest exercise routine you possibly can. It's much better to find the one that is best suited to your own goals and condition. Some vigorous exercise programs may very well *not* be for you. All things considered, it may be wiser and more enjoyable to stick with a lighter workout than to risk injury or burnout by pursuing too aggressive a routine. With that thought in mind, let's briefly consider some ideas for more vigorous exercise programs.

Some exercise activities are moderately vigorous. They can be boosted up to a more vigorous level if they are done briskly or for longer periods. Examples include calisthenics, singles tennis, and volleyball.

More vigorous exercises are desirable for people who are capable of them because such exercises condition the heart and lungs if done properly. These activities use the large muscles of the body. They need to be done at a level of high intensity for at least half an hour. They also need to be done on a regular basis, three or four times a week.

Examples of these include aerobic dancing, brisk walking, cross-country skiing, and hiking uphill. They also include jogging, jumping rope, rowing, running in place, stationary cycling, and swimming. All of these can provide good workouts—but only for those who get their doctor's approval to pursue them.

Pace Yourself

You should enjoy the exercise program you choose. There is no need—ever—to knock yourself out or exercise above a comfortable pace in order to get some benefit from the activity. Remember to stop any exercise if you feel pain, discomfort, or fatigue. Build up your stamina slowly. It may even take a few weeks of exercising before you start to feel the results. Stay with it! Check yourself as you go. If you can do the following, you are probably working out at the appropriate level.

- Speak comfortably. As you exercise, you should be able to carry on a conversation easily with others.
- Feel fine after you stop exercising. You should be back to normal within ten minutes of stopping.

If you have a hard time breathing, feel faint, or are very weak after exercising, you are working too hard. Cut back on your intensity for a while.

Almost everyone misses some exercise sessions because of illness. If that happens to you, wait until you feel healthy again before going back to your workouts. Similarly, if you become injured, wait until you are healed and the pain is gone before starting again. If you do have to miss some workouts, start again at a lower level. Then slowly work back up to where you were before.

You'll want to go easy with your exercise program in the beginning. Plan to reach your long-term exercise goals slowly but surely. Don't expect to exercise at maximum intensity for a sustained period during the very first week of your program. Instead, work up to that goal gradually, over a number of weeks or even months. Your body will let you know when to push harder and when to lay off a little bit.

A structured workout program should follow a bell-shaped activity curve. Start out slowly, with gentle stretching and warm-up activities that last about five minutes. Gradually build your intensity. For maximum cardiovascular benefit, you may work out at a level plateau for between thirty minutes and an hour. (Stretching and relaxation exercises may not last that long.) After that, gradually taper off in your movements and cool down. End by repeating the gentle stretching exercises you began with.

Bear in mind that if you have exercised vigorously for at least half an hour, you have maximized your cardiovascular benefits for that session. Some benefit occurs with lesser amounts of exercise. Continued effort beyond thirty minutes does not yield further benefit to your heart and lungs (although you will continue to burn calories at a higher rate). Use common sense and keep your activities enjoyable. Listen to your body for any sign that you may be working too long or too hard, and slow down if necessary.

Avoid Injuries

Some people are leery of starting a personal exercise program because they fear being injured. Exercise always carries some risk of injury. But the risks don't have to be great, especially if you take sensible precautions. Prevention is still the best medicine where injuries from exercise are concerned. Remember to avoid exercising too hard at the beginning of your program. Also, if you ever feel winded, faint, or ill while exercising, slow down or stop. Take your time. The following precautions can help you avoid exercise injuries.

1. Use the proper equipment for your activity. If you walk, for example, that means wearing good shoes that support your feet and ankles and provide plenty of cushioning. If you do stretching exercises and have a balance problem, it means using a sturdy chair with armrests for support, or a seat belt if you are in a wheelchair. You may need to have someone on hand to assist you in some movements. Investigate what you may need before you start a program.

2. Build up your activity level gradually. Warm up before each exercise session to prevent cramps and sprains in involved limbs and joints. With vigorous exercise, give yourself time to reach your target intensity level. After working at your desired level of intensity, slowly taper off. Do "cooling down" stretching exercises before stopping completely. This will help prevent muscle cramping.

3. Listen to your body. Overexertion can injure you. If you become too tired, you can make mistakes more easily. You may trip or twist an ankle as a result. You can also put too much wear and tear on your body. This applies to any activity with repetitive motions and to vigorous exercise. Pay attention to any early warning pains that develop in the joints, feet, ankles,

or legs—or anywhere else. Stop the activity immediately, and don't start again until the pain is completely gone. Continuing to exercise when you feel joint or muscle pain risks injuring those areas much more seriously.

4. Be aware of signs of possible heart problems. Occasionally, people have died from cardiac arrest while exercising. While the risk of cardiac arrest goes up slightly during exercise, the overall risk of an arrest is greatly decreased in people who are active. There are some precautions that can help assure you a healthy, enjoyable exercise period. Get an evaluation from your doctor before you start your own program. Again, don't start exercising until you have brought a high blood pressure condition down to normal range. You may be having heart problems if you feel a sudden pain or pressure develop in your mid-chest area or on the left side of the neck, shoulder, or arm during or just after exercising. This may be accompanied by a sudden lightheadedness. Your face may become pale, and you may break out in a cold sweat. If these symptoms happen to you, stop exercising immediately and seek a doctor's help.

   Note: The chest pain described here is different from that of a so-called **side stitch.** A side stitch is a fairly common, temporary condition in which a sudden cramp develops below the rib cage of a person who is exercising vigorously.

5. Take account of the weather and time of day. Different weather conditions can pose different risks. Sunrise and twilight can impair your visibility and that of others who may be sharing the road with you. If you walk outdoors as your exercise program, you'll need to adjust to these conditions. (Consider an alternative, indoor activity for those days when you just don't feel like tackling snow or humidity.)

On hot and humid days:

- Walk during the cooler part of day.
- Walk less than normal until you acclimate.
- Drink plenty of fluids, especially water.
- Wear a minimum of light, loose clothing. Wear light colors that reflect sunlight away from your body. Wearing a sun hat and sunglasses is a good idea.
- Don't wear very stretchy or tight, rubberized clothing. Don't wear sweat pants or sweatshirts. They retain heat and can cause dangerously high body temperatures. Some people wear sweats because they believe that doing so helps them lose weight faster. This isn't true. The water you lose by sweating is quickly replaced in the body when you drink water.

On cold days:

- Wear several layers of clothes—one layer less than you would wear if you weren't going to be exercising.
- Protect your hands with gloves or mittens.
- Wear a hat. Forty percent of your body heat can escape through your uncovered neck and head.

In rain, ice, or snow:

- Be aware of reduced visibility—your own and others'. This can also be a problem at dawn or dusk, when there is less natural light. Stay on sidewalks and out of the road wherever possible.
- Take special care to walk slowly and carefully.

How to Enjoy Exercise for Life

While your exercise routine is still new, anticipating the eventual benefits can be hard. That can make it difficult to maintain your commitment. If you are finding it hard to keep your exercise program on track, try these tips.

1. Set your sights on short-term as well as long-term goals. Start with an exercise goal that is less ambitious than your ultimate goal. For example, if you

eventually want to be able to walk for forty-five minutes at a time, concentrate on working up to a twenty-
minute walk first. Then gradually add extra minutes
until you have reached your long-term goal.

2. Discuss your goals with family and friends. Their support will strengthen your resolve. And they may even
decide to join you.

3. If you're having trouble sticking to your plan, list the
benefits of the activity and refer to the list often. (See
page 264, which discusses some of these benefits.)

4. If you don't like your chosen exercise program, try to
evaluate why. First, try to find out why you are bored
or frustrated by your activity. Then you will be in a
better position to pick a new one that you will like
better and stick with.

The right exercise plan for you doesn't have to be competitive,
exhausting, or unpleasant to get you into better shape. As we've
seen, a good program can take many appealing forms and still
achieve your most important goal—personal fitness. Work with
your doctor to set up a program that is right for you. You'll find
that regular exercise is a truly enjoyable activity—literally, the
experience of a lifetime.

Stress

A lot of attention has been focused recently on the effect of
stress on human health. No proven relationship links high
stress with stroke. However, feelings of sustained stress and anxiety
may lead to other behaviors that are more directly linked to stroke
risk, such as smoking and high blood pressure.

Stress cannot always be avoided, but it can be managed. For
stroke survivors, a lot of stress can be alleviated just by knowing
what to expect from their illness or the therapies they are following.
If you feel uncertain about any part of your treatment program, be
sure to ask plenty of questions and get the answers you need.

Stressed-out people need to learn to recognize when they are becoming tense and anxious. At those times, it helps to divert one's attention in some way from what is upsetting. Some people have had success with a behavior modification technique called the "relaxation response." The idea is to interrupt tense, stressful feelings and replace them with quieter, soothing ones. There are other ways to short-circuit those feelings and become calmer, too. Regular exercise can help, and so can meditation. Some people are soothed by a gentle massage. Consult your doctor, or investigate books on this subject in your library.

The Stroke Prevention Equation: Evaluation Plus Effort

As this book tries to show, there is a lot you can do to reduce the risk of having a first or second stroke. So much has been learned in the past twenty years alone! Today we know more than ever before about what causes stroke and how to treat it. New drugs and new diagnostic tests will continue to be developed in the future.

But equally important, we are learning to appreciate just how significant our daily habits are to lifelong health. Lifestyle adjustments have everything to do with personal health. They can be large or small. They can involve what we eat and how much exercise we get. They can involve decisions about whether or not we monitor medical conditions like high blood pressure, and whether or not we smoke. They cannot in themselves provoke or prevent stroke, of course. Other unchangeable factors, including one's heredity, are also involved.

Yet making an effort to live every day as healthfully as possible can certainly help reduce your chance of having a stroke. You can start with some of the guidelines discussed here. With that effort, a doctor's evaluation and guidance, and the support of family and friends, you can make a positive change in your life.

Appendix A

The American Heart Association Diet: An Eating Plan for Healthy Americans

Goals of the AHA Eating Plan

Reducing your "controllable" risk factors—those you can change—may help prevent a stroke in the future.

Heart disease is one of the major risk factors for stroke. High blood cholesterol is one of the major risk factors for heart disease. Better food habits can help you reduce high blood cholesterol. This eating plan from the American Heart Association describes the latest advice of medical and nutrition experts. The best way to help lower your blood cholesterol level is to eat less saturated fatty acids and cholesterol, and control your weight. The AHA Diet gives you an easy-to-follow guide to eating, with your heart and brain in mind.

The eating plan is based on these AHA dietary guidelines:

- Total fat intake should be less than 30 percent of calories.
- Saturated fatty acid intake should be less than 10 percent of calories.
- Polyunsaturated fatty acid intake should be no more than 10 percent of calories.
- Monounsaturated fatty acids make up the rest of total fat intake, about 10 to 15 percent of total calories.
- Cholesterol intake should be no more than 300 milligrams per day.
- Sodium intake should be no more than 3,000 milligrams (3 grams) per day.

How Can I Use This Plan?

This section lists the basic food groups. It gives you the number of servings per day from each food group, serving sizes, and some suggested food choices. It's important to select a variety of foods within each food group. This section also lists desserts, snacks, and beverages you may choose.

If you eat the *lower* number of servings from each food group, you will get enough protein, vitamins, and minerals—nutrients that your body needs each day. Eat moderate amounts of foods from the meat, fish, poultry, egg, and fat groups. You may choose more servings of foods from the other groups if you don't need to lose weight or if you wish to gain weight.

The American Heart Association suggests this plan for all healthy Americans two years of age and older. Slight modifications may be necessary for growing children and teenagers. You must be sure they get enough energy (calories) and nutrients each day. If you or others in your family are pregnant or breast-feeding, or have a medical disorder such as diabetes, talk to your doctor, a registered dietitian, or a licensed dietitian or nutritionist about your special dietary needs.

Eating Plan Tips

To control the amount and kind of fat, saturated fatty acids, and dietary cholesterol you eat:

- Eat no more than 6 *ounces* (cooked) per day of lean meat, fish, and skinless poultry.
- Try main dishes featuring pasta, rice, beans, and/or vegetables. Or create "low-meat" dishes by mixing these foods with small amounts of lean meat, poultry, or fish.
- The approximately 5- to 8-teaspoon servings of fats and oils per day may be used for cooking and baking, and in salad dressings and spreads.
- Use cooking methods that require little or no fat—

boil, broil, bake, roast, poach, steam, sauté, stir-fry, or microwave.

- Trim off the fat you can see before cooking meat and poultry. Drain off all fat after browning. Chill soups and stews after cooking so you can remove the hardened fat from the top.
- The 3 to 4 egg yolks per week included in your eating plan may be used alone or in cooking and baking (including store-bought products).
- Limit your use of organ meats, such as liver, brains, chitterlings, kidney, heart, gizzard, sweetbreads, and pork maws.
- Choose skim (nonfat) or 1% fat milk and nonfat or low-fat yogurt and cheeses.

To round out the rest of your eating plan:

- Eat 5 or more servings of fruits or vegetables per day.
- Eat 6 or more servings of breads, cereals, or grains per day.

Meat, Poultry, and Fish
High in Protein, B Vitamins, and Iron and Other Minerals

Servings per day:
No more than 6 ounces cooked lean meat, poultry, and fish
Serving size:
3 ounces cooked (4 ounces raw) lean meat, poultry, or fish
Here are some examples to help you judge serving sizes of meat, poultry, and fish. A 3-ounce portion equals:

- the size of a deck of playing cards
- 2 thin slices of lean roast beef (each slice 3" x 3" x ¼")
- ½ of a chicken breast or a chicken leg with thigh (without skin)
- ¾ cup of flaked fish

Choose from:
Fish—fresh, frozen, canned in water (or rinsed)

Shellfish*
Chicken (without skin)
Cornish hen (without skin)
Turkey (without skin)
Turkey, ground
Lean beef** (from the round, sirloin, loin)
Lean or extra-lean ground beef
Lean ham†
Lean pork (tenderloin, loin chop)
Lamb (except rib)
Veal (except commercially ground)
Wild game‡—rabbit, venison, pheasant, duck (without skin)

- Organ meats are very high in cholesterol. However, liver is rich in iron and vitamins, and a small serving (3 ounces) is okay about once a month.
- Trim off all the fat before cooking meat. Drain or skim off fat from cooked meats before using juices in stews, soups, gravies, etc.
- Remove the skin and fat under the skin from poultry pieces before cooking. If you're roasting a whole chicken or turkey, leave the skin on to keep the bird from getting too dry while roasting. Then remove the skin before carving and serving the meat.
- Select whole turkeys that have not been injected with fats or broths.
- Frozen dinners and entrees may also fit into the plan. **Look for those that are made specially for low-fat, low-cholesterol, low-sodium diets.**
- A one-cup serving of cooked beans, peas, or lentils, or 3 ounces of soybean curd (tofu) can replace a 3-ounce serving of meat, poultry, or fish.

---

* Shrimp and crayfish are higher in cholesterol than most other types of fish, but lower in fat and cholesterol than most meats and poultry.
** Buy "choice" or "select" grades of beef rather than "prime."
† Ham and Canadian bacon are higher in sodium than other meats.
‡ Domesticated versions of game (duck and goose) are not as lean as wild game.

Eggs
High in Protein, B Vitamins, and Iron and Other Minerals

Servings per week:
3 to 4 egg yolks a *week* may be eaten (egg whites are not limited)

- Because of their cholesterol content (213 milligrams per yolk), limit your whole eggs and egg yolks to no more than 3 to 4 per week. Be sure to count any egg yolks used in cooking and in store-bought foods in your total for the week.
- Use two egg whites, or one egg white plus 2 teaspoons of unsaturated oil, in place of one whole egg in cooking. You can also use cholesterol-free commercial egg substitutes.
- Eat only *cooked* eggs and egg whites—not raw.

Vegetables and Fruits
High in Vitamins, Minerals, and Fiber; Low in Fat, Calories, and Sodium; Contain NO Cholesterol

Servings per day:
5 or more
Serving size:
1 medium-size piece of fruit or ½ cup fruit juice
½–1 cup cooked or raw vegetables
Choose often: All vegetables and fruits except coconut. Olives and avocados should be counted as fats (see "Fats and Oils" section). Starchy vegetables are listed with "Breads, Cereals, Pasta, and Starchy Vegetables" because they are similar in calories per serving to the other foods in that group.

- Enjoy plenty of fruits and vegetables. These foods will give you vitamins, minerals, and fiber with few calories. Be sure to include sources rich in vitamin C and vitamin A.
- Check the labels for sodium content of canned vegetables.

Milk Products
High in Protein, Calcium, Phosphorus, Niacin, Riboflavin,
Vitamins A and D

Servings per day:
2 or more for adults over 24 years and children 2–10 years
3–4 for ages 11–24 and women who are pregnant or breast-
feeding
Serving size:
1 cup skim, ½% or 1% fat milk
1 cup nonfat or low-fat yogurt
1 ounce low-fat cheese or ½ cup low-fat cottage cheese
Choose from:
Milk products with 0–1% fat:
skim milk
½–1% fat milk
nonfat or low-fat dry milk powder
evaporated skim milk
buttermilk made from skim or 1% fat milk
nonfat or low-fat yogurt
drinks made with skim or 1% fat milk and cocoa (or other low-
fat drink powders)
Low-fat cheeses:
dry-curd, skim, or low-fat cottage cheese
natural or processed cheeses with no more than 5 grams of fat
per ounce

- Skim, ½% fat, and 1% fat milk all provide the same
  nutrients as whole milk and 2% fat milk. But they are
  much lower in fat, saturated fatty acids, cholesterol,
  and calories.
- If you're used to whole milk products, you may find it
  easier to make the change slowly to lower-fat foods.
  Try 2% fat milk first. Then when you're used to that,
  move to 1% fat milk. That will make it much easier if
  you decide to change to skim milk.

Breads, Cereals, Pasta, and Starchy Vegetables
Low in Fat and Cholesterol; High in B Vitamins, Iron, and Fiber

Servings per day:
6 or more
Serving size:
1 slice bread
1/4 cup nugget or bud-type cereal
1/2 cup hot cereal
1 cup flaked cereal
1 cup cooked rice or pasta
1/4–1/2 cup starchy vegetables
1 cup low-fat soup
Choose from the following examples of available foods in this group:

Breads and rolls
wheat, rye, raisin, or white bread
English muffins
frankfurter and hamburger buns
water (not egg) bagels
pita bread
tortillas (not fried)

Crackers and snacks*
animal, graham, rye crackers
soda, saltine, oyster crackers
matzo
fig bar, gingersnap, molasses cookies
bread sticks, melba toast
rusks, flat bread
pretzels (unsalted)
popcorn (see "Fats and Oils" for preparation)

Quick breads**
homemade using margarine or oils low in saturated fatty acids,
skim or 1% fat milk, and egg whites or egg substitutes (or egg
yolks within limits)
biscuits, muffins, cornbread

---

* Many kinds of crackers and snacks are now available with no added salt or unsalted tops. Some are high in saturated fatty acids, so read the labels.
** If you use any egg yolks in cooking quick breads, be sure to count them in your daily allowance.

fruit breads, soft rolls

pancakes, French toast, waffles

Hot or cold cereals†

all kinds (granola-type may be high in fat or saturated fatty acids)

Rice and pasta†

all kinds (pasta made without egg yolk)

Starchy vegetables

potatoes, corn

lima beans, green peas

winter squash

yams, sweet potatoes

Soups‡

chicken noodle

tomato-based seafood

chowders

minestrone

onion

split pea

Fats and Oils

Some of these foods are high in vitamins A or E, but all are high in fat and calories.

Servings per day:

No more than a total of 5–8, depending on your caloric needs

Serving size:

1 teaspoon vegetable oil or regular margarine

2 teaspoons diet margarine

1 tablespoon salad dressing

2 teaspoons mayonnaise or peanut butter

3 teaspoons seeds or nuts

⅛ of medium avocado

10 small or 5 large olives

---

† Cereals, pasta, and rice cooked without salt are lower in sodium than instant or ready-to-eat types of these foods.

‡ Most soups are high in sodium and some are high in fat. When buying soups, read labels and choose those low in sodium and fat. You can also make your own soups and control both sodium and fat.

Choose from:

Vegetable oils and margarines with no more than 2 grams of saturated fatty acids per tablespoon—canola, corn, olive, safflower, sesame, soybean, sunflower.

Salad dressings and mayonnaise with no more than 1 gram of saturated fatty acids per tablespoon.

- Use fats and oils sparingly—and use the ones lowest in saturated fatty acids and cholesterol.
- Use hydrogenated shortenings sparingly and choose those made from vegetable fat. They are lower in saturated fatty acids than those made from animal/vegetable fat blends.
- Use cooking styles that add little or no fat to food, and ask for them when eating out.
- Remember to count the "hidden fat" in bakery and snack foods, as well as the fats used in cooking and on vegetables and breads.
- Remember that although coconut oil, palm oil, and palm kernel oil are vegetable oils and have no cholesterol, they are high in saturated fatty acids. *Read food labels carefully.*

Desserts

Choose:

Desserts low in saturated fatty acids, cholesterol, and calories. For a special treat, share a dessert portion with someone.

First Choices (low in fat and saturated fatty acids):

Fruit—fresh, frozen, canned, or dried

Low-fat yogurt with fruit

Crackers and cookies (as listed in the "Breads, Cereals, Pasta, and Starchy Vegetables" section)

Angel food cake

Frozen low-fat or nonfat yogurt

Sherbet or ice milk

Flavored gelatin

Water ices or sorbet

Special Occasions Only (higher in fat and calories):
   Homemade desserts (cakes, pies, cookies, puddings)—made with margarine or oils low in saturated fatty acids, skim or 1% fat milk, and egg whites or egg substitutes (or egg yolks within limits).
   Store-bought desserts—many are now made with unsaturated oils and are either low-fat or nonfat. Be sure to read ingredient lists.

Snacks

Choose snacks from other food groups, such as:
   Fruits and juices
   Raw vegetables and low-fat dips
   Low-fat cookies
   Low-fat crackers
   Plain unsalted popcorn
   Unsalted pretzels
   Hard candy, gumdrops
   Sugar, syrup, honey, jam, jelly, marmalade (as spreads)

Beverages

First Choices:
   Fruit or vegetable juice, coffee, tea, plain or flavored mineral water, low-sodium broth, and low-sodium bouillon
Other Choices:
   Fruit punches, carbonated soft drinks
   Alcoholic beverages: If you drink them, do so in moderation. Have no more than two drinks per day of wine, beer, or liquor, and only when caloric limits allow. Here are the amounts to count as *one* drink (½ ounce pure alcohol):

12 ounces	Beer
1½ ounces	80-proof spirits (bourbon, gin, rum, Scotch, tequila, vodka, whiskey)
1 ounce	100-proof spirits
4 ounces	Wine (red, white, rosé)

   If you don't drink, don't start!

For More Information

For help in changing your recipes to fit this plan, you may find the *American Heart Association Cookbook: Fifth Edition* useful. More tips for dining out and preparing food are in the *American Heart Association Low-Fat, Low-Cholesterol Cookbook*. You'll find low-fat recipes that are also low in sodium in the *American Heart Association Low-Salt Cookbook*. All of these are available in your local bookstores.

The *American Heart Association Fat and Cholesterol Counter* lists the fat, saturated fatty acid, cholesterol, sodium, and calorie content of more than 450 common foods. You can find it in bookstores and grocery stores. For more information about nutrition, diet, and heart disease, contact your nearest American Heart Association.

Appendix B

For Further Information

Note: Listed below are organizations, companies, books, periodicals, and videocassettes that may provide information of interest to stroke survivors and their families. Inclusion in this list does not constitute an endorsement, implied or otherwise, by the American Heart Association.

Organizations

The organizations listed below offer information and educational materials for stroke survivors and their families. Some may refer inquiries to chapter offices, local agencies, or local resources that provide certain services.

General Information

American Heart Association National Center
7272 Greenville Avenue
Dallas, TX 75231-4596
(800) AHA-USA-1
(See list of AHA Affiliates, pages 308–309.)

Stroke Connection
A Service of the American Heart Association
7272 Greenville Avenue
Dallas, TX 75231-4596
(800) 553-6321

National Council on the Aging, Inc.
409 Third Street, SW
Second Floor
Washington, DC 20024
(202) 479-1200

National Easter Seal Society
70 East Lake Street
Chicago, IL 60601
(800) 221-6827

National Health Information Center
Office of Disease Prevention and Health Promotion
U.S. Public Health Service
Department of Health and Human Services
PO Box 1133
Washington, DC 20013-1133
(800) 336-4797

National Stroke Association
8480 East Orchard Road
Suite 1000
Englewood, CO 80111-5015
(303) 771-1700

Stroke Connection
A Service of the American Heart Association
7272 Greenville Avenue
Dallas, TX 75231-4596
(800) 553-6321

Well Spouse Foundation
PO Box 28876
San Diego, CA 92198-0876
(619) 673-9043

Diet, Rehabilitation, and Travel Information

American Dietetic Association
216 West Jackson Boulevard
Suite 800
Chicago, IL 60606-6995
(312) 899-0040

American Health Care Association
1201 L Street, NW
Washington, DC 20005-4014
(202) 842-8444

American Occupational Therapy Association
1383 Piccard Drive
PO Box 1725
Rockville, MD 20850-0822
(301) 948-9626

American Physical Therapy Association
1111 North Fairfax Street
Alexandria, VA 22314-1488
(703) 684-2782

American Speech-Language-Hearing Association
10801 Rockville Pike
Rockville, MD 20852
(800) 638-8255

National Aphasia Association
Murray Hill Station
PO Box 1887
New York, NY 10156-0611
(800) 922-4622

National Association of Social Workers
750 First Street, NE
Suite 700
Washington, DC 20002
(800) 638-8799

National Institute on Deafness and Other
   Communication Disorders
Building 31, Room 3C-35
National Institutes of Health
9000 Rockville Pike
Bethesda, MD 20892
(301) 496-7243

Society for the Advancement of Travel for the Handicapped
347 Fifth Avenue
Suite 610
New York, NY 10016
(212) 447-7284

Visiting Nurse Associations of America
3801 East Florida Avenue
Suite 900
Denver, CO 80210
(800) 426-2547

Local Resources

State Department on Aging
State Vocational Rehabilitation Agencies
Local Health Departments
Veterans Administration Hospitals

Fulfilling Special Needs

Each company listed below offers a full line of easy-to-use clothing available for sale to the general public. Call or write for a free catalog or to order clothing.

J.C. Penney Company
PO Box 65900
Dallas, TX 75265-9000
(214) 431-3816

Patient's Personal Needs, Inc.
275 Centre Street
Holbrook, MA 02343
(800) 289-4776

Wardrobe Wagon, Inc.
555 Valley Road
West Orange, NJ 07052
(800) 992-2737

Books

The following books may be available from your local bookstore, library, or stroke support group. Some may also be ordered directly from the publisher.

American Heart Association. *American Heart Association Fat and Cholesterol Counter.* New York: Times Books, 1991.

American Heart Association. *The One-Handed Way.* Dallas: American Heart Association, 1993.

Ancowitz, Arthur, M.D. *The Stroke Book.* New York: William Morrow and Company, Inc., 1993.

Bell, Lorna, R.N., and Eudora Seyfer. *Gentle Yoga.* Berkeley: Celestial Arts, 1987.

Cole, Harry A. *Helpmates: Support in Times of Critical Illness.* Louisville, Kentucky: Westminster/John Knox Press, 1991.

Gordon, Neil F., M.D., Ph.D., MPH. *Stroke: Your Complete Exercise Guide.* Champaign, IL: Human Kinetics Publishers, 1993.

Grundy, Scott M., M.D., Ph.D., and Mary Winston, Ed.D., R.D., eds. *American Heart Association Low-Fat, Low-Cholesterol Cookbook.* New York: Times Books, 1989.

Legato, Marianne J., M.D., and Carol Colman. *The Female Heart: The Truth about Women and Coronary Artery Disease.* New York: Simon & Schuster, 1991.

Murphy, Jo. *Keys to Fitness Over 50.* New York: Barron's, 1991.

Paullin, Ellen. *Ted's Stroke: The Caregiver's Story.* Cabin John, Maryland: Seven Locks Press, 1988.

Shimberg, Elaine F. *Strokes: What Families Should Know.* New York: Ballantine Books, 1990.

Starke, Rodman D., M.D., and Mary Winston, Ed.D., R.D., eds. *American Heart Association Low-Salt Cookbook.* New York: Times Books, 1990.

Winston, Mary, Ed.D., R.D., ed. *American Heart Association Cookbook,* Fifth Edition. New York: Times Books, 1991.

Zaret, Barry L., M.D., et al., eds. *Yale University School of Medicine Heart Book.* New York: Hearst Books, 1992.

Zemach-Bersin, David, et al. *Relaxercise.* San Francisco: Harper Collins, 1990.

Periodicals

The following newsletter is written by and for stroke survivors and their families. For information on other newsletters, contact your local stroke club or the American Heart Association's Stroke Connection (page 290).

Stroke Connection. Published six times a year by the American Heart Association's Stroke Connection, 7272 Greenville Avenue, Dallas, TX 75231-4596.

Videocassette Tapes

The following tapes may be available from your local American Heart Association, hospital, library, or stroke support group. Some may also be ordered directly from the company or association listed.

The Healing Influence: Guidelines for Stroke Families. Dana Evans Balibrera, Danamar Productions, Santa Fe, New Mexico, 1990.

Moving Easy: Lift-Free Patient Transfers. Frank Hatch, Lenny Maietta, and Dana Evans Balibrera, Danamar Productions, Santa Fe, New Mexico, 1993.

Stroke. Churchill Films, Inc., Los Angeles, California, 1983.

Stroke: Focus on Feelings. Oracle Film & Video, Santa Monica, California, 1986.

Stroke: Focus on the Family. Oracle Film & Video, Santa Monica, California, 1988.

A Stroke Survivor's Workout. American Heart Association's Stroke Connection, Dallas, Texas, 1988.

Glossary

Abnormal glucose tolerance The inability to metabolize sugar in the diet properly.

Abulia A neurologic disorder that is caused by brain damage and is marked by the loss of will or interest.

Acute Severe, but of short duration, as opposed to chronic.

ADLs (activities of daily living) Common activities of everyday life.

Agnosia The inability to comprehend sensory information. A person with agnosia, for example, may ignore everything on the left side of his body even though there is no dysfunction of vision and hearing on that side. In this case, the condition is the result of a stroke on the right parietal lobe of the cerebrum.

Agraphia The inability to express thoughts in writing because of a brain injury.

Alexia The inability to read because of a brain injury.

Aneurysm A ballooning-out of the wall of a blood vessel, usually an artery, or of the heart due to weakening of the wall by disease, injury, or an abnormality present at birth.

Angiography (arteriography) A diagnostic technique in which a dye is injected into selected blood vessels, which are then photographed using X rays. Angiography can give a good idea of the condition of veins and arteries and alert doctors to the presence of blood clots.

Anomia The inability to name objects or people.

Anosognosia A condition in which a person seems to be unaware of or indifferent to his disabilities.

Anticoagulant An agent that prevents blood from clotting.

Aphasia Language problems caused by damage to the brain. People with aphasia may have trouble speaking, understanding, writing, or reading.

Arrhythmia An abnormal heart rhythm.

Arteriovenous malformation (AVM) A congenital condition in which arteries directly connect with veins. These areas of connection are thin-walled and apt to leak. AVMs are frequently associated with subarachnoid hemorrhage.

Artery Any one of a series of blood vessels that carry blood from the heart to the various parts of the body. Arteries have thick, elastic walls that can expand as blood flows through them.

Ataxia Muscular incoordination, especially regarding gait (walking).

Atherosclerosis A form of artery disease in which the inner layers of artery walls become thick and irregular because of deposits of cholesterol and other substances. As the interior walls of arteries become lined with layers of these deposits, the arteries become narrowed, and the flow of blood through them is reduced. This buildup, **atheroma,** is sometimes called **plaque.** Some people refer to atherosclerosis as "hardening of the arteries."

Atrial fibrillation The rapid, uncoordinated contractions of individual heart muscle fibers in the upper chambers of the heart. These chambers, called the atria, can't contract in a coordinated fashion, and they pump blood ineffectively, if at all.

Blood clot A jelly-like mass of blood tissue formed by clotting factors in the blood. This clot can then stop the flow of blood from an injury. Blood clots also can form inside an artery whose walls are damaged by atherosclerotic buildup and can cause a heart attack or stroke.

Brain hemorrhage Uncontrolled bleeding in or on the brain.

Brain stem The part of the brain located at the top of the spinal cord and extending up to the midbrain area.

Broca's aphasia A disorder in which the person has difficulty speaking and making himself understood. He knows what he wishes to say, but because of his brain injury, cannot find the words. The person with Broca's aphasia often speaks in short bursts and repeats words. Also called expressive aphasia, motor aphasia, and nonfluent aphasia.

Bruits Abnormal sounds or murmurs heard over blood vessels. Pronounced "broo-EE."

Calcium channel blockers A type of drug that acts to stop excessive amounts of calcium from collecting in the cells and triggering other damaging chemical reactions. Calcium channel blockers are useful for some heart patients, but their use is still experimental for stroke patients.

Capillary   Microscopically small blood vessel between arteries and veins that allows exchange of oxygen and other nutrients between the blood and body tissues.

Cardiac   Pertaining to the heart.

Cardiovascular disease   Disease of the heart and blood vessels, including stroke, rheumatic heart disease, and high blood pressure.

Caregiver   Any person who provides the primary care to a sick or injured person. May be a family member, friend, or professional.

Carotid artery   A major artery in the neck carrying blood to the brain.

Carotid endarterectomy   Surgical removal of plaque deposits or blood clots in the carotid arteries.

Central nervous system   The part of the nervous system made up of the brain and the spinal cord.

Cerebellum   The part of the brain that is concerned with coordinating voluntary movements, balance, and posture. The cerebellum is located at the back of the brain, below the cerebrum.

Cerebral cortex   The heavily wrinkled outer layer of the cerebrum. Composed of nerve cells, the cerebral cortex is where much of human reasoning and complicated voluntary movements occurs. Also called **gray matter.**

Cerebral embolism   A blood clot formed in one part of the body and then carried by the bloodstream to the brain, where it lodges in an artery.

Cerebral hemorrhage   Bleeding within the brain, resulting from a ruptured aneurysm or a head injury.

Cerebral thrombosis   Formation of a blood clot in an artery that supplies part of the brain.

Cerebrospinal fluid (CSF)   The fluid in which the brain sits inside the skull.

Cerebrovascular occlusion   The obstruction or closing of a blood vessel in the brain.

Cerebrum   The largest part of the brain. Divided into two halves, or hemispheres, the cerebrum is where voluntary movements originate and where thought processes are coordinated.

Cholesterol   A fatlike substance found in animal tissue. Cholesterol is present only in foods from animal sources, such as dairy products, meat, fish, poultry, animal fats, and egg yolks.

Chronic   Having a long duration, as opposed to **acute.**

Circulatory system   Pertaining to the heart, the blood vessels, and the circulation of blood.

Collateral blood flow   A system of smaller arteries, closed under normal circumstances, that may open up and start to carry blood to part of the brain when a cerebral artery is blocked. Over a long period of time, new vessels may grow into poorly supplied areas. Both sets of events can serve as alternative routes of blood supply.

Computed tomography (CT scan, CAT scan)   An important test for evaluating brain tissue. A CT scan can usually identify whether a stroke was due to bleeding or a blockage.

Congenital   Refers to a condition present in the body at birth.

Congestive heart failure   The inability of the heart to pump out all the blood that returns to it. This results in blood backing up in the veins that lead to the heart and sometimes in fluid accumulating in various parts of the body.

Conjugate gaze paralysis   A condition in which the patient's eyes are frozen to one side.

Deficit   Another term for a physical or cognitive disability.

Diabetes mellitus (diabetes)   A disease in which the body doesn't produce or properly use insulin. Insulin is needed to convert sugar and starch into the energy needed in daily life. Diabetes increases the risk of developing cardiovascular disease.

Diastolic blood pressure   The lowest blood pressure measurement in the arteries. It occurs when the heart muscle is relaxed between beats.

Diuretic   A drug that promotes the excretion of water and salts, increasing the rate at which urine forms.

Dominant   In human biology, the slightly more developed element of a pair, as in "his left hand was slightly dominant compared to his right."

Dysarthria   The imperfect articulation of speech, sometimes resulting from muscular problems caused by damage to the brain or nervous system.

Dysphagia   Difficulty in swallowing or inability to swallow. This condition has a variety of causes, including brain damage or physical injury to the face, mouth, neck, or throat areas.

Edema   Swelling due to an abnormally large amount of fluid in body tissues.

Electrocardiogram (EKG or ECG)   A graphic record of electrical impulses produced by the heart.

Embolic stroke   Occurs when a brain artery is blocked by a clot that has formed elsewhere—usually in the heart or neck arteries—and been carried through the bloodstream to the brain.

Embolus   A blood clot that forms in a blood vessel in one part of the body and then is carried to another part of the body. Plural is *emboli.*

Fibrin   A protein in the blood that enmeshes blood cells and other substances during blood clotting. Fibrin creates the substantial part of the blood clot. Fibrin is formed from fibrinogen.

Frozen shoulder   A painful, avoidable condition in which an impaired shoulder becomes stiff with disuse and at risk of becoming dislocated. Frozen shoulder can be avoided with gentle range-of-motion exercises started soon after a stroke.

Gray matter   Same as **cerebral cortex.**

Heart attack   Death of, or damage to, part of the heart muscle due to an insufficient blood supply. Also known as **myocardial infarction.**

Hematoma   A swelling filled with excess blood.

Hemianopia   Partial blindness caused by damage to the brain. The person's vision is "blacked out" in the left or right visual field of both eyes.

Hemiplegia   Paralysis of one side of the body.

Hemorrhage   Profuse bleeding from a ruptured blood vessel.

Heparin   A type of anticoagulant drug that prevents clotting by affecting the blood component fibrinogen.

High blood pressure   A chronic increase in blood pressure above its normal range. Blood pressure is considered high when a reading of 140/90 or greater is measured on several successive occasions. High blood pressure increases the risk of heart disease and kidney disease and is a major risk factor for stroke. The technical term for high blood pressure is **hypertension.**

High-density lipoprotein (HDL)   A carrier of cholesterol believed to transport cholesterol away from the tissues and to the liver, where it can be excreted. Sometimes called the "good cholesterol," in comparison to low-density lipoprotein (LDL).

Hypertension   Same as **high blood pressure.**

Hypoperfusion The inability of the vascular system to supply an outlying arterial area with blood, commonly due to a lack of blood pressure or an arterial blockage.

Hypothalamus The small part of the brain that coordinates many functions of the central nervous system, including sex drive, hunger, and thirst.

Infarction Death of tissue due to a lack of blood, usually caused by a blockage in an associated artery.

Intracerebral hemorrhage (ICH) Occurs when an artery deep in the brain ruptures and blood pressing into the brain tissue destroys it.

Ischemia Decreased blood flow to an organ, usually due to constriction or obstruction of an artery.

Lacune A small cavity in the substance of the brain. The hole is believed to be caused by the death of tissue during a **transient ischemic attack.**

Lipid A fatty substance insoluble in blood.

Lipoprotein The combination of lipid surrounded by a protein; the protein makes it soluble in blood.

Low-density lipoprotein (LDL) The main carrier of harmful cholesterol in the blood. Called the "bad cholesterol," in comparison to high-density lipoprotein (HDL).

Lumbar puncture An invasive test in which a sample of cerebrospinal fluid is taken from a needle inserted in the spinal column. The fluid is then analyzed for evidence of subarachnoid hemorrhage or other unusual causes of stroke. Sometimes called a **spinal tap.**

Lumen The inner part of a tube, such as a blood vessel.

Magnetic resonance imaging (MRI) A noninvasive diagnostic tool for examining the brain and other parts of the body. Using a magnetic field, MRI excites atoms within that field with radio waves and then uses a computer to pick up the signals that the atoms throw off. The computer translates these signals into a picture image of the part of the body under observation.

Medulla Part of the brain stem that controls breathing, among other things.

Midbrain Part of the brain stem.

302

Middle cerebral artery (MCA)   A major artery of the brain that supplies most of the upper brain. Each cerebral hemisphere is supplied by an MCA.

Monounsaturated fat   A type of fat found in many foods but predominantly in canola, olive, and peanut oil, and avocados.

Myocardial infarction   The damaging or death of an area of the heart muscle (myocardium) resulting from a reduced blood supply to that area. Also known as **heart attack.**

Neglect   A neurologic disorder in which the patient ignores one side of his body, half of his visual field, or both. Usually a result of a stroke on the right hemisphere of the brain and affecting the left side of the body.

Neurologist   A physician who specializes in diagnosing and treating diseases of the brain and other parts of the nervous system.

Neurons   The basic cell unit of the nervous system. Neurons send and receive electrical impulses between the brain and the rest of the body.

Neutropenia   A disorder in which the blood lacks the usual number of infection-fighting white cells.

Obesity   The condition of being significantly overweight, usually 30 percent or more over ideal body weight. Obesity puts a strain on the heart and can increase the chance of developing high blood pressure and diabetes.

Occlusion   Occurs when something such as a blood clot, or thrombus, blocks a blood vessel completely.

Occupational therapist   A health care professional certified to teach people who have had a stroke or other injury to become as independent as possible in their daily activities at home, on the job, and in the community.

Parietal lobe   The part of the brain in which spatial orientation is coordinated. It is located in the back part of the head, behind the frontal lobe and above the temporal lobe.

Peripheral nervous system   A collection of nerves that fan outward from the spinal column to reach every part of the body.

Physical therapist A health care professional certified to teach people who have had a stroke or other injury to become as independent as possible in large motor activities, such as rolling over in bed, walking, or using a wheelchair.

Plaque Also called atheroma, this is a deposit of fatty and other substances in the inner lining of the artery wall. It is characteristic of atherosclerosis.

Platelet antiaggregant/platelet inhibitor A class of drugs that prevent platelets from sticking together and clotting the blood. Aspirin and ticlopidine are common examples of platelet antiaggregants.

Platelets One of the three kinds of formed elements found in the blood, platelets aid in the clotting of the blood.

Polycythemia A "thick blood" condition in which too many red blood cells are present in the blood. Polycythemia can aggravate an atherosclerotic condition and increase the risk of stroke.

Polyunsaturated fats Oils of vegetable origin, such as corn, safflower, sunflower, and soybean oils, that are liquid at room temperature.

Pons Part of the brain stem that links the back of the brain to the upper portions, allowing them to communicate with each other.

Primary risk factor Risk factor that directly affects the risk of stroke. High blood pressure, heart disease, cigarette smoking, previous stroke, age, sex, race, diabetes mellitus, and transient ischemic attacks (TIAs) are primary risk factors for stroke.

Psychologist A health care professional certified to diagnose emotional problems and disorders of higher function of the nervous system. As part of a stroke team, psychologists help patients and their families deal with emotional problems caused by disability.

Rehabilitation Process of restoring lost or impaired functions (e.g., walking, communicating) to the highest level that can be achieved after a stroke or other injury.

Rehabilitation team The group of specialists who work together to provide people with the medical care, therapy, counseling, and family training needed to recover from an illness or injury. Members of a stroke rehab team may include the stroke survivor, his or her family, medical specialists, dietitian/nutritionist, rehabilitation nurse, physical therapist, occupational therapist, speech therapist, recreational therapist, social worker, and psychologists.

Rheumatic heart disease Damage done to the heart, particularly the heart valves, by one or more attacks of rheumatic fever.

Risk factor When referring to the heart and blood vessels, a risk factor is associated with an increased chance of developing cardiovascular disease, including stroke. Some risk factors are genetic, some are the product of natural processes, and some are the result of personal lifestyle.

Saturated fats Types of fat found in foods of animal origin and a few of vegetable origin. They are typically solid at room temperature.

Secondary risk factor Risk factor that indirectly affects the risk of stroke because it increases the risk of heart disease or other primary risk factors for stroke. Obesity, high blood cholesterol levels, and excessive alcohol drinking are secondary risk factors for stroke.

Social worker A health care professional certified to help patients and their families adjust to problems caused by illness and disability, including insurance and financial problems.

Sodium A mineral essential to life, sodium is found in nearly all plant and animal tissue. Table salt (sodium chloride) is nearly half sodium.

Spasticity A condition in which limb muscles abnormally contract, causing exaggerated reflexes and increased resistance to stretching.

Spatial awareness The ability to organize objects in relation to one another, as in judging distance.

Speech and language specialist A health care professional trained to identify, test, diagnose, and treat people with speech, language, voice, stuttering, and/or swallowing disorders.

Sphygmomanometer An instrument for measuring blood pressure.

Spinal tap See **Lumbar puncture.**

Stenosis The narrowing or constriction of an opening, such as a blood vessel.

Stress Bodily or mental tension within a person resulting from his or her response to physical, chemical, or emotional factors. Stress can refer to physical exertion as well as mental anxiety.

Stroke The sudden interruption of the blood supply to the brain, caused either by a blockage or a rupture of blood vessels. Older terms for stroke include apoplexy and cerebrovascular accident (CVA).

Stroke belt An eleven-state area in the southeastern U.S. with a higher-than-average incidence of stroke. The states included are: Alabama,

Arkansas, Georgia, Indiana, Kentucky, Louisiana, Mississippi, North Carolina, South Carolina, Tennessee, and Virginia.

Subarachnoid hemorrhage (SAH)   Occurs when there is uncontrolled bleeding on the surface of the brain in the area between the brain and the skull.

Systolic blood pressure   The highest blood pressure measured in the arteries. It occurs when the heart contracts with each heartbeat.

Thrombocytosis   A disorder in which an unusually large number of thrombocytes are in the blood. Thrombocytes are blood platelets that play a role in blood clotting.

Thrombolysis   The breaking up of a blood clot.

Thrombolytic agents   Drugs that work by dissolving blood clots in arteries.

Thrombotic stroke   A stroke caused by a blood clot, or **thrombus,** that forms in an artery going to the brain. The clot blocks the passage of blood to a part of the brain.

Thrombus   A blood clot that forms inside a blood vessel or cavity of the heart.

Tissue plasminogen activator (t-PA)   A natural protein that works by dissolving blood clots in arteries, restoring blood flow. Currently t-PA is used for heart patients, but is considered an experimental therapy for stroke patients. Also called a "clot buster."

Transcranial Doppler ultrasound (TCD)   A noninvasive diagnostic test that uses ultrasound techniques to generate information about affected intracranial blood vessels. TCD helps doctors precisely to locate atherosclerosis in the intracranial arteries and to determine the extent of the damage.

Transient ischemic attack (TIA)   A very small stroke that is caused by a temporarily blocked blood vessel and leaves no permanent brain damage. Symptoms for TIA are the same as for a stroke but are temporary, usually lasting twenty-four hours or less. TIAs are an important warning sign of an impending stroke and should never be ignored. Prompt medical attention could prevent a full-blown stroke from occurring.

Triglyceride   The chemical form in which most fats exist in the blood. High triglyceride levels often accompany high overall blood cholesterol levels and are associated with the risk of developing diabetes.

Ultrasound   High-frequency sound vibrations, not audible to the human ear, used in medical diagnoses, such as **transcranial Doppler ultrasound** tests (TCDs).

Vascular   Pertaining to the blood vessels.

Vasoconstriction   A spasm in which the vessel lumen narrows dramatically and reduces the area through which blood may pass.

Vein   Any one of a series of blood vessels of the vascular system that carries blood from various parts of the body back to the heart.

Vertebral artery   One of two such arteries in the neck that supply the back of the brain with blood. Halfway up the neck, these arteries become entwined with the neck vertebrae before entering the head.

Warfarin   A synthetic anticoagulant that works by preventing certain blood clotting agents from forming in the liver.

Warning signs of stroke   Symptoms that indicate that a stroke may be imminent. Medical attention must be sought as soon as possible after the warning signs have been observed.

The warning signs of stroke are:
Sudden weakness or numbness of the face, arm, or leg on one side of the body
Sudden dimness or loss of vision, particularly in one eye
Loss of speech, or trouble talking or understanding speech
Sudden, severe headaches with no apparent cause
Unexplained dizziness, unsteadiness, or sudden falls, especially along with any of the previous symptoms

Wernicke's aphasia   A disorder due to brain damage in which the patient loses the ability to understand the spoken or written word. A person with Wernicke's aphasia may talk a lot but often doesn't make sense. Also called receptive aphasia, fluent aphasia, sensory aphasia.

White matter   The inner substance of the brain, composed mostly of nerve fibers that transmit the impulses generated by nerve cells (**gray matter**) on the **cerebral cortex.**

American Heart Association Affiliates

American Heart Association National Center, Dallas TX

AHA, Alabama Affiliate, Inc., Birmingham, AL

AHA, Alaska Affiliate, Inc., Anchorage, AK

AHA, Arizona Affiliate, Inc., Phoenix, AZ

AHA, Arkansas Affiliate, Inc., Little Rock, AR

AHA, California Affiliate, Inc., Burlingame, CA

AHA of Metropolitan Chicago, Inc., Chicago, IL

AHA of Colorado, Inc., Denver, CO

AHA, Connecticut Affiliate, Inc., Wallingford, CT

AHA, Dakota Affiliate, Inc., Jamestown, ND

AHA of Delaware, Inc., Newark, DE

AHA, Florida Affiliate, Inc., St. Petersburg, FL

AHA, Georgia Affiliate, Inc., Marietta, GA

AHA, Hawaii Affiliate, Inc., Honolulu, HI

AHA of Idaho, Inc., Boise, ID

AHA, Illinois Affiliate, Inc., Springfield, IL

AHA, Indiana Affiliate, Inc., Indianapolis, IN

AHA, Iowa Affiliate, Inc., Des Moines, IA

AHA, Kansas Affiliate, Inc., Topeka, KS

AHA, Kentucky Affiliate, Inc., Louisville, KY

AHA, Greater Los Angeles Affiliate, Inc., Los Angeles, CA

AHA, Louisiana, Inc., Destrehan, LA

AHA, Maine Affiliate, Inc., Augusta, ME

AHA, Maryland Affiliate, Inc., Baltimore, MD

AHA, Massachusetts Affiliate, Inc., Framingham, MA

AHA of Michigan, Inc., Lathrup Village, MI

AHA, Minnesota Affiliate, Inc., Minneapolis, MN

AHA, Mississippi Affiliate, Inc., Jackson, MS

AHA, Missouri Affiliate, Inc., St. Louis, MO

AHA, Montana Affiliate, Inc., Great Falls, MT

AHA, Nation's Capital Affiliate, Inc., Washington, DC

AHA, Nebraska Affiliate, Inc., Omaha, NE

AHA, Nevada Affiliate, Inc., Las Vegas, NV

AHA, New Hampshire Affiliate, Inc., Manchester, NH

AHA, New Jersey Affiliate, Inc., North Brunswick, NJ

AHA, New Mexico Affiliate, Inc., Albuquerque, NM

AHA, New York City Affiliate, Inc., New York City, NY

AHA, New York State Affiliate, Inc., North Syracuse, NY

AHA, North Carolina Affiliate, Inc., Chapel Hill, NC

AHA, Ohio Affiliate, Inc., Columbus, OH

AHA, Northeast Ohio Affiliate, Inc., Cleveland, OH

AHA, Oklahoma Affiliate, Inc., Oklahoma City, OK

AHA, Oregon Affiliate, Inc., Portland, OR

AHA, Southeastern Pennsylvania Affiliate, Inc., Philadelphia, PA

AHA, Pennsylvania Affiliate, Inc., Camp Hill, PA

Puerto Rico Heart Association, Inc., Hato Rey, Puerto Rico

AHA, Rhode Island Affiliate, Inc., Pawtucket, RI

AHA, South Carolina Affiliate, Inc., Columbia, SC

AHA, Tennessee Affiliate, Inc., Nashville, TN

AHA, Texas Affiliate, Inc., Austin, TX

AHA, Utah Affiliate, Inc., Salt Lake City, UT

AHA, Vermont Affiliate, Inc., Williston, VT

AHA, Virginia Affiliate, Inc., Glen Allen, VA

AHA, Washington Affiliate, Inc., Seattle, WA

AHA, West Virginia Affiliate, Inc., Charleston, WV

AHA, Wisconsin Affiliate, Inc., Milwaukee, WI

AHA of Wyoming, Inc., Cheyenne, WY

Index